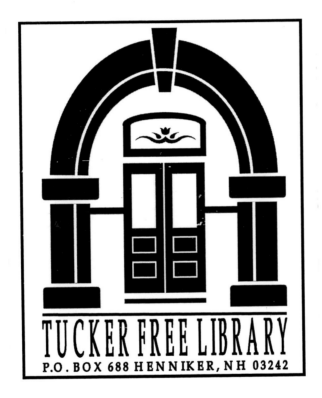

Cook for Your Life

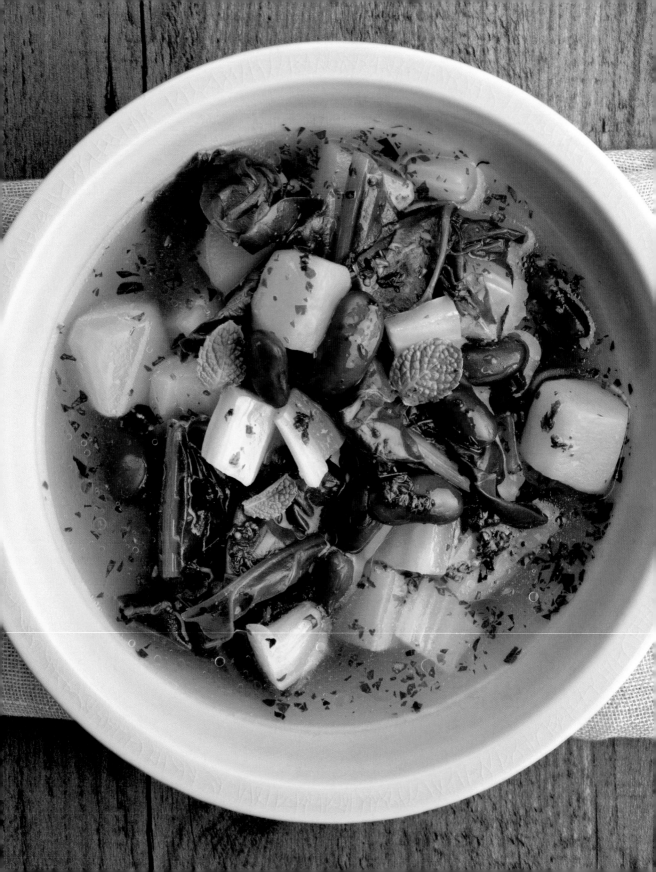

Cook for Your Life

· · · · · · · · ❧ · · · · · · · ·

DELICIOUS, NOURISHING RECIPES
FOR BEFORE, DURING, AND AFTER
CANCER TREATMENT

Ann Ogden Gaffney

AVERY

an imprint of Penguin Random House

New York

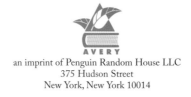

an imprint of Penguin Random House LLC
375 Hudson Street
New York, New York 10014

Most Avery books are available at special quantity discounts for bulk purchase for sales promotions, premiums, fund-raising, and educational needs. Special books or book excerpts also can be created to fit specific needs. For details, write SpecialMarkets@penguinrandomhouse.com.

Library of Congress Cataloging-in-Publication Data

Gaffney, Ann Ogden.
Cook for your life : delicious, nourishing recipes for before, during, and
after cancer treatment / Ann Ogden Gaffney.
p.   cm.
Summary: "A beautiful, unique cookbook with delicious recipes for all stages of cancer treatment and recovery, from a two-time cancer survivor and founder of the Cook for Your Life nutrition-based cooking programs"—Provided by publisher.
Includes bibliographical references and index.
ISBN 978-1-58333-581-9 (hardback)
1. Cancer—Diet therapy.   2. Cancer—Diet therapy—Recipes.   I. Title.
RC271.D52G34   2015   2015014773
641.5'631—dc23

Printed in the United States of America
1   3   5   7   9   10   8   6   4   2

Book design by Meighan Cavanaugh

For anyone who has ever received a cancer diagnosis and wondered

how they are ever going to cope with eating and nourishing

themselves or a loved one through the hardships of cancer treatment.

This cookbook is dedicated to you.

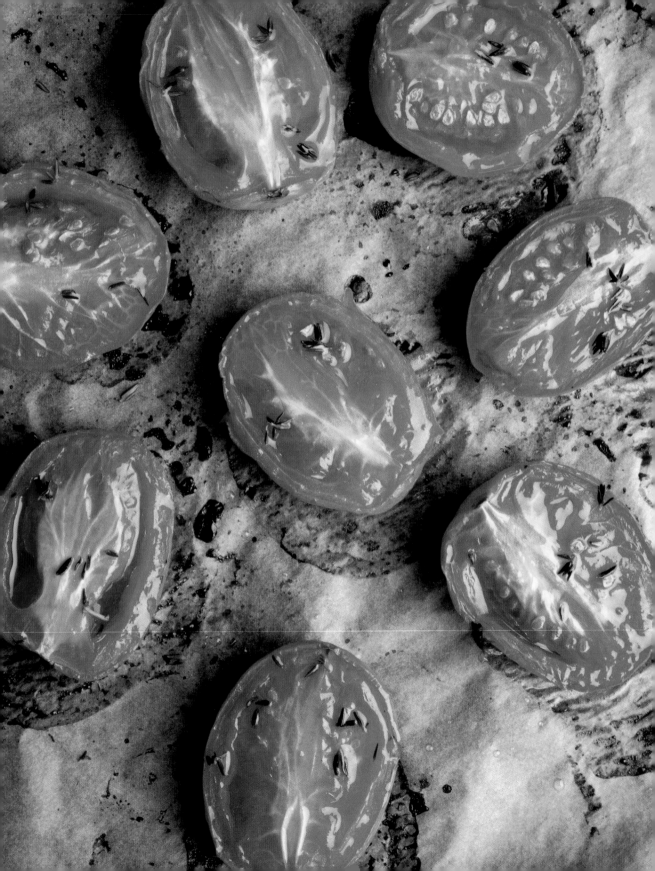

Contents

· · · ✦ · · ·

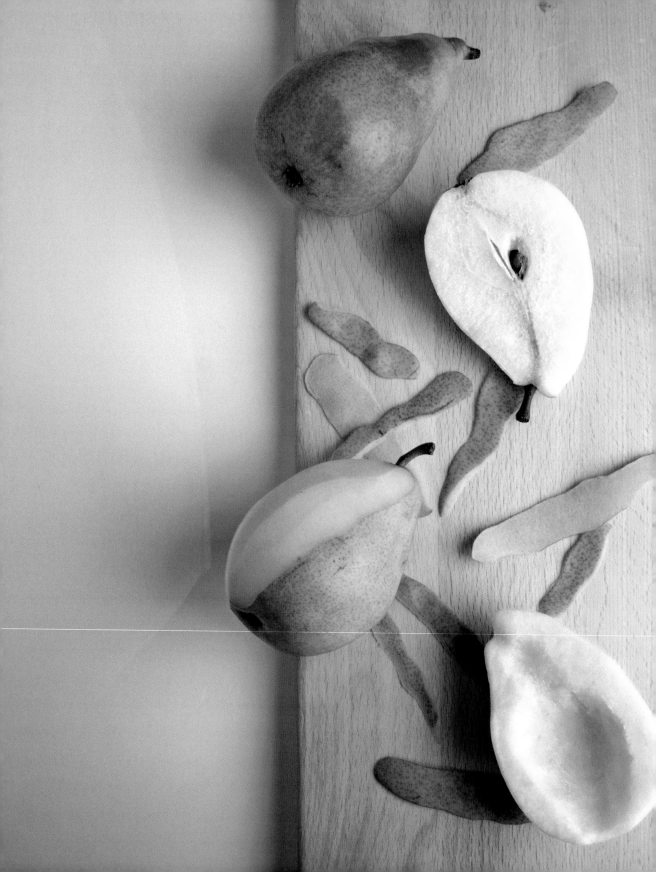

Acknowledgments

Getting this book together has been an amazing experience that could not have happened without not just a little, but a lot of help from my friends.

First of all, I would like to thank the Cook for Your Life team: my fabulous board chair, Nancy Rutter Clark, whose friendship, support, and belief in our mission have helped bring CFYL to where it is today; my friend Bruce Crouch, CFYL's first benefactor, who loaned me his kitchen, gave me his time, and shared his love of cooking with me to help with the initial testing of my recipe ideas; Chelsea Fisher, my right-hand woman, whose creativity, palate, organizational skills, and knowledge of CFYL's DNA were crucial in helping me pull all the threads of this book together; Joe Gaffney, my darling husband and amazing photographer, who put up with not only me throughout the whole process (he deserves sainthood) but with talented chef and food stylist extraordinaire Mariko Makino, who created the beautiful images in this book on our dining room table—thank you both from the bottom of my heart; Ty Donald, who helped us get the manuscript ready, and Angie Marin, whose support on CFYL's teaching side gave me the space to get the book finished. Thank you.

To the others who gave their valuable time to this book: Alex Rothwell, RD, CSO, CDN, who read through each recipe to verify its nutrition info; Anne Wright, who edited the recipes to make sure they were ready for the publisher; and Dr. Stewart

Fleischman, an early believer in CFYL, who wrote the wonderful foreword. Thank you. Thank you.

This list would not be complete without my wonderful editor, Lucia Watson, who helped me every step of the way.

And very special thanks to my agent, Judy Linden, whose relentless belief in this book made me a believer, too.

The recipes in a cookbook have to work. A shout-out to friends across the country who took the time to test the raw recipes in their home kitchens so we could work out any kinks—Alexis Quinlan: your baking prowess rules. Ed Machado: the best notes! Spider Fawke: I'd wait impatiently each morning for your snaps of the food and your comments. Janet Waddell: The girl who doesn't cook cooked! Mark Welsh and James Salaiz: I loved how you two just jumped into that cake. Dr. Heather Greenlee: my partner in crime at Columbia University's Mailman School of Public Health who found time to try things out for us. Sam Osborn, who, with Chelsea Fisher, tested the recipes on their unsuspecting friends. Katie Fisher: queen of all things spicy. Gaby Longhi Chautin: my fish wrangler. Susan Morningstar: beet dominatrix. And not forgetting Ty Donald, Angie Marin, Joe Fazio, and Chef Seppo Ed Farrey. Last but not least, Dr. Jon Deutsch of Drexel University and his team at the Food Lab led by Ally Zeitz. Thank you all.

And to my friends, family, and colleagues whose friendship, love, and encouragement have helped me along the CFYL way: Gaye Sandler and Roger Miller; Simon Doonan and Jonathan Adler; Louise Crandall; Jenny Capitain; John Bird; Esther Trepal, RN, MS, CDN; Bridget Bennett, MS, RD; Robert Forrest; Harlan Bratcher and Toby Usnik; Cydney Cort; Clive Rigby; Chris Spencer and Kim Swink; Letty Simon; Suleika Jaouad; John Rossi; Colleen Roche; Seigan Ed Glassing; Delphine Blue; Kerry Warn; Freddie Lieba; Ellen Scordato; Dr. Martha Eddy; Stephen Malamud, MD; Stefanie Saks, MS, CNS, CDN; Robin Osler and Bruce Matthews; James Morales; Karen Hibma; Edward Sherman; Becky Klein, Keith Klein, Sarah Bird; Billy Kent; Ruth Fehr; Chris Dewey; Robert Shepherd; Governor Christie Whitman; Richard and Jane Ogden; Frank and Katie Ogden; Johnny O'Green; Dr. Susan Teeger; Rodrigue Le Van Hyunh; Johnno Duplessis; Chef Naxielly Dominguez; Chef Dylana Deganes; Owen Edwards; and last the CFYL board: Your guidance and unwavering support have been invaluable to me.

Love and special thanks to Rene Taylor, who, as our hair grew back and life beckoned again, lit the fire under me that made this new journey seem possible.

In memoriam: To those I wish I could proudly share this book with—my mum and dad, Adrian Cartmel, Kathy Russell Rich, Michael Cronan, Joan Deignan, Roberta Van Laven, Tom Hadder, Hans the herring king, Ann Craig, Chayo Mata, Dr. Steven Tamarin, and Christine Zounek. I miss you.

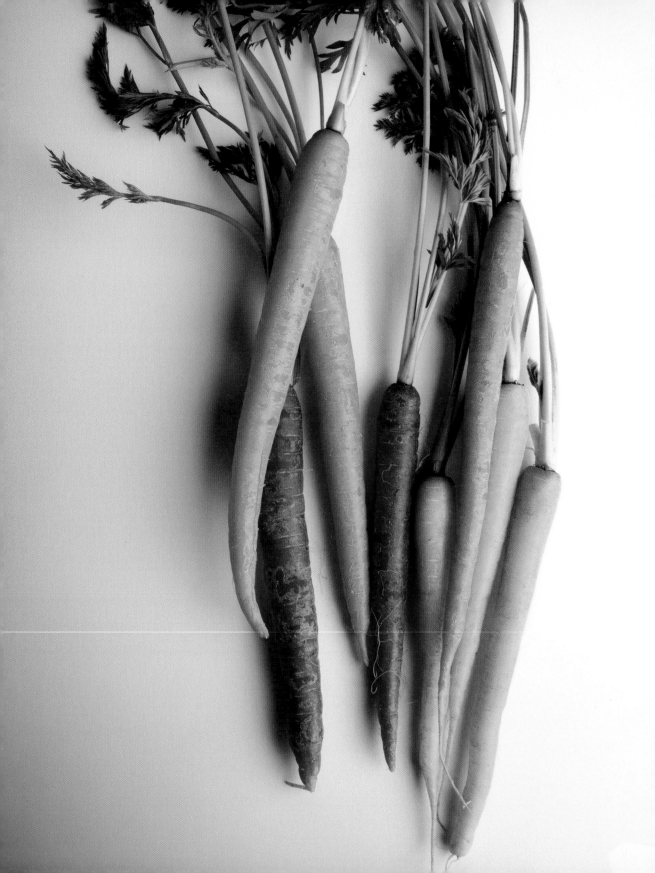

Foreword

Good food is one of the most underestimated elements of successful cancer treatment. The ill effects both of cancer and its therapies—fatigue, loss of lean body mass, infection, and blood-clotting difficulties, to name just a few—can be positively influenced by optimal nutrition. Though supplements are widely available as canned drinks, capsules, or tablets, food's beneficial and enjoyable properties need not be simulated when they are found at their best, in nature's original packaging. Most of us connect healthy eating with cancer prevention, but much less attention is paid to the importance of appealing foods during or after chemotherapy, radiation, or surgery.

Cook for Your Life is *not* your usual cookbook. Rather than being organized around meal types or biochemical categories, this wonderful book celebrates our primordial attachment to food: simple, soothing, safe, sweet, and scrumptious. The science stands behind the food rather than as its calling card.

When cancer cells grow and multiply quickly, they use an extraordinary amount of energy, estimated to be in the many thousands of calories each day. That is far more energy than is supplied by even a calorie-rich diet, causing a deficit that a specially designed diet has to address. The increased *quantity* of calories needs to be from *good* sources: deeply colored vegetables and fruits, whole grains, low-fat proteins, and monounsaturated fats—all necessary components to maintain one's energy levels and bodily functions. When appetite is curtailed and fear grows, we often reach for our comfort foods, and *Cook for Your Life* shows how those can be both delicious and reparative.

Whether you are an experienced chef or need coaching for anything more complicated than reheating leftovers, this book can teach and motivate. With time between doctor appointments, chemotherapy, radiation, periods of recovering from surgery, learning a few basic cooking techniques is a welcome diversion as well as a practical guide to food as a potent recuperative approach. Appetite changes and difficulties with taste, smell, or even swallowing have tried-and-true workarounds with properly prepared high-quality foods. Ann Ogden has channeled her personal experiences as a cancer survivor, her professional skills as a chef, and her experience as a master teacher to bring this information to you and your supportive family and friends.

In every culture, food brings us together. That effect of community is never more necessary than when someone is facing cancer. To strive for the best and longest survivorship, let *Cook for Your Life* guide you to better eating, more energy, and an improved quality of life, whether you are at the start of treatment, in the middle of the journey, or beyond. This unique book gives special meaning to the wish offered by chefs through the ages: Bon appétit!

—*Stewart B. Fleishman, MD,*
Founding Director, Cancer Supportive Services,
Mount Sinai Health System

Cook for Your Life

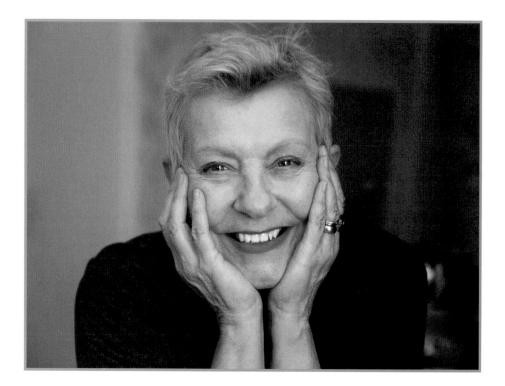

My Story

If you'd told me ten years ago I'd be a leader in the world of culinary medical initiative, collaborating on programs with Columbia University and backed by data and studies funded by the National Institutes of Health (NIH), and a published academic researcher, I would have asked you what you were smoking. And yet, that is what happened.

I was a fully paid-up member of the glamorous world of fashion. I'd started out as a painter, and while at art school I made clothes, both for myself and for friends. This morphed into a career in fashion after an editor at British *Vogue* spotted one of my jackets at a party and introduced me into the London fashion scene. A year later, I was scouted for a job in Paris, and I moved there intending to stay six months. I stayed twelve years. I worked for some of the top names of the time, including couturier Hubert de Givenchy. In 1985, I moved to New York City, where I became a design consultant for industry giants like Calvin Klein, J.Crew, Saks, and Barneys.

My fashion career allowed me to indulge in two personal passions: food and travel. I come from a family of foodies and world travelers. Dad was a master baker, and on Mom's side, all Italians, both my grandfather and uncle were chefs.

I first traveled abroad at age eight and began cooking at twelve, learning Italian specialties from my mom's side of the family and sturdy British classics from my dad's. Wherever I traveled as an adult—and in fashion that meant often and worldwide—I steeped myself in the local cuisines. These new flavors eventually made their way into my cooking.

During the years when AIDS decimated the fashion community, I cooked and cared for one of my oldest friends during the last six months of his life. This guy was amazing. He lived until he simply couldn't be himself anymore. In the process, he taught me not to be afraid. The experience changed me. I didn't realize how much until years later while on my cancer journey.

I was first diagnosed with cancer after a routine ob-gyn checkup in fall 2001. It had completely taken over my right kidney. I was lucky. I had surgery to remove the offending organ and life went back to the normal routine of work and travel. Three and a half years later, it was a different story. My second diagnosis was an unrelated triple-negative breast cancer that would require surgery, chemo, and radiation. I'd just finished a big project. I knew I wouldn't be able to travel and doubted I would have the energy to give the 110 percent needed to start something new. And I would be bald. I decided to take a hiatus from work and to give myself the time and space to get through my treatment.

This decision changed my life. Taking that step back helped me to connect with my new reality. As I became immersed in the world of hospitals and cancer treatment, I began to understand how my cooking skills were helping me to cope with my side effects better than my fellow travelers on the cancer road. Cooking allowed me to adjust to taste changes and adapt my food to how I was feeling at any given moment. One day, while listening to a friend at a support group describe her problems with food and taste, I realized that the hospital staff was giving her information on alleviating her symptoms but couldn't help her put this advice into action. That's when I knew I could help. My love of food and cooking had given me the tools to deal with my own treatment side effects, and my experience as a caregiver to my friend with AIDS had taught me the importance of nourishment and the sheer comfort good food could bring during illness. I started to offer advice, then recipes, and then I organized free cooking classes. I loved it.

When my treatment finally ended, I took a meeting with a client to talk about a new fashion project. As I sat listening to the talk of color and trends, I realized that my heart was no longer in it. I didn't want to get back into endless discussions about a shade of blue or skirt lengths. I wanted to go back to the people in the cancer suite who so badly needed help to cook and eat better.

I didn't take the job. In 2007, I founded Cook for Your Life.

Since that time, Cook for Your Life has gone from a one-woman show to a thriving nonprofit organization that is a leader in the growing field of the culinary medical initiative. It has directly served more than seven thousand New Yorkers and has a peer-reviewed and published National Cancer Institute–funded research program in collaboration with Columbia University's Mailman School of Public Health, as well as an interactive recipe website that serves more than one hundred thousand patients and their families each month.

This success has been built on the relaxed, caring atmosphere of our classes. Working together in the warmth of a kitchen helps people to build confidence, share support, and learn skills that get good nutrition onto their plates and good eating habits into their lives. It also empowers. At a time when patients' lives are ruled by their medical teams, our classes are geared toward giving them back control over one major aspect of their lives: food. With this cookbook, I hope to bring into your own kitchen the warmth, joy, and delicious food we make at our classes.

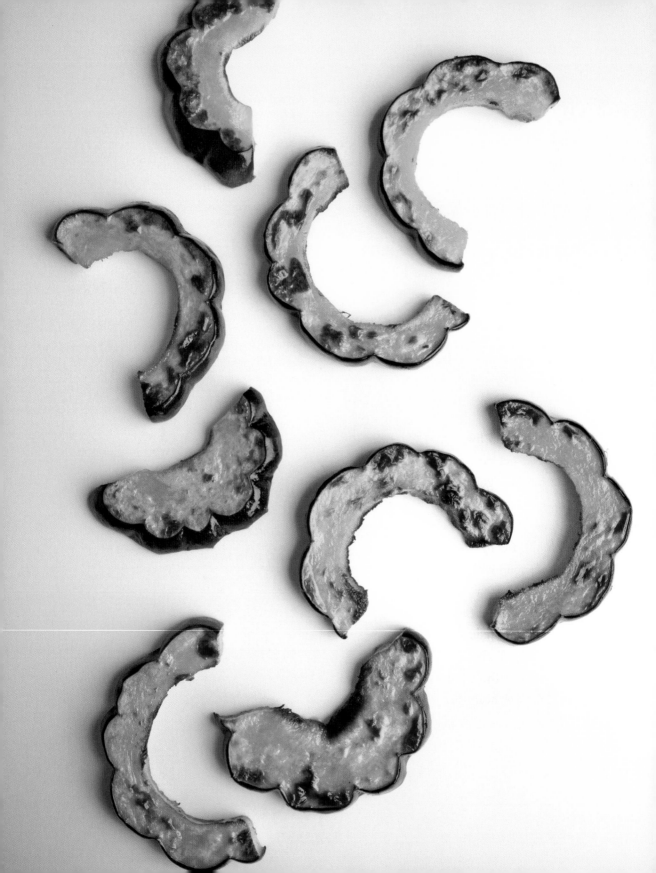

Sidelining the Side Effects

I love to cook and I live to eat. Two cancer diagnoses couldn't put a dent in that, but they did get me thinking about food.

When I was going through chemo and radiation for my second cancer, a well-meaning friend who knew of my love of all things edible sent me two cancer-themed cookbooks to help me along on my journey. One was written by a nutritionist and the other by a doctor. Great, I thought. I opened the first book randomly to a recipe for soup with a huge list of ingredients to prep. The second book was similarly complex, with recipes that were dull and uninspiring. Both books were well-intentioned, but clearly neither author had experienced the mind-numbing fatigue of chemo or radiation or the vagaries of damaged taste buds. The thought of shopping for and chopping all those vegetables was more than my limited energy could cope with. The books were relegated to the shelf, and I returned to cooking the simple, healthy food I'd been making all along—food that felt right for me and my body.

I am grateful to these two books. Their shortcomings gave me an insight that has proved invaluable. When you have cancer, cooking isn't just about healthy eating; it is also about feelings, both physical and mental.

Cancer treatment protocols have their ups and downs, bringing good days and bad, and although each day is different, a rhythm starts to build that allows you to predict when you're going to feel your worst or be at your best. Good food can help you get through all of it. It can soothe or it can excite. It can certainly make you feel human again.

And, of course, good food is delicious food. I dislike the attitude of deprivation and faddishness attached to the idea of healthy eating. I've been around long enough to see eggs both vilified and lauded, butter banned from our tables then grudgingly invited back. And so it goes. To my mind, good food is never about what you can't have; it's always about what you can.

During the often arduous cancer journey, cooking also gives you control. When cancer forced me to hand my body over to my medical team, I found that cooking for myself and my family gave me a positive path back into life after doctors: At least I could control the food I put into my body. Many of the people who come to Cook for Your Life classes feel the same way. And cooking can bring a rush of instant gratification at a time when it feels as if you're always waiting for something, whether for test or CAT scan results, or your doctor, or simply for the grueling months of treatment to be over. Cooking a meal that gives you healthy deliciousness in minutes equals control over an important part of your life.

I wanted the layout of this book to reflect and connect with how it feels as you work your way through the different phases of treatment. To give you what you need, the recipes are organized into the chapters "Simple," "Soothing," "Safe," "Spicy," "Sweet," and "Scrumptious." On the days during chemo and radiation when you feel at your exhausted, nauseated worst, or hormone therapy has sucked up all your energy, go to "Simple" or "Soothing." On the days when life is all but back to normal and you just want to enjoy feeling better and being alive, tuck into the recipes of "Safe," "Spicy," or "Sweet." And I haven't forgotten healthy survivor-ship, either. "Scrumptious" is there for that. It is essential. There are more than eighteen million of us in the United States either living with cancer or having survived it. I want to help us all to eat better, stay well, fight cancer with our forks, and **to cook for our lives**.

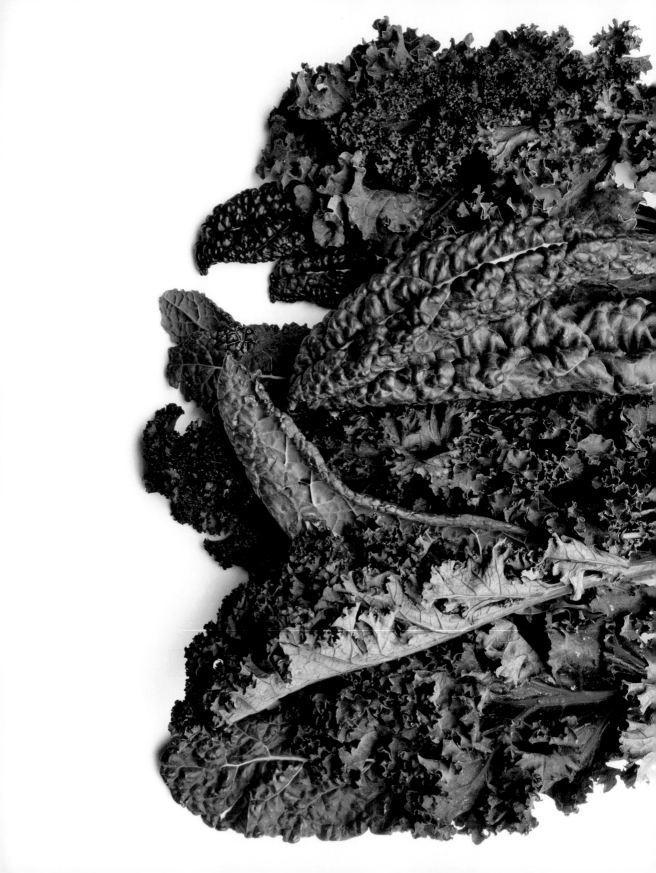

How to Use This Book

In each recipe you'll find boxed text titled "Ann's Tips." These are some of my tried-and-true tricks in the kitchen as well as ingredient replacements or adjustments you may need or want to make. There are also "Health Tips" to give you useful information about ingredients and help with problems of treatment.

"Health Considerations" and "Food Preferences" appear at the beginning of each recipe, as they apply. These are to help you navigate any of the special diets or dietary recommendations you may have been given by your doctor or registered oncology dietician (a glossary of terms follows).

HEALTH CONSIDERATIONS

This is a guide to the way the recipes are labeled for quick reference. For example, if your doctor has put you on a bland or a neutropenic (antimicrobial) diet, the appropriate recipes are grouped under those headings. Or if you want recipes specific to being in treatment, there are recipes listed under that, too. And there are also recipes listed under specific side effects like nausea or fatigue. All the recipes in this book are in the 400-calories-and-under range per portion, so if you need to up your calories, increase your intake of healthy oils, like olive oil, or healthy fatty foods, like avocado.

And for those of you who want to search by ingredient, food preference, or health consideration, you will find the recipes pinpointed in the index at the end of the book.

Here is a glossary of terms.

IN TREATMENT

These recipes contain important nutrients needed to maintain strength throughout chemotherapy, radiation, and/or surgery recovery. They tend to contain comforting, cooked foods. As chemo affects everyone's tastes a bit differently, the options range from easy-to-digest to hot and spicy.

FATIGUE

Fatigue is, sadly, a necessary evil of many treatment protocols. While there is no "magic" food to combat these feelings of exhaustion, our recipes offer easy, comforting options for when you may be too tired to prepare a complex meal. Although sugary treats will pick you up temporarily, excess amounts of refined carbohydrates can increase feelings of lethargy once the initial burst of energy wears off, so the foods in this category tend to be lower in starches. As a side note, one of the proven aids for fatigue is exercise! It seems counterintuitive, but moving can provide energy, helping one feel less tired. Getting off the couch and into the kitchen to prepare a simple meal will not only nourish you but could lift your spirits as well!

EASY TO SWALLOW

A side effect of some chemo drugs is painful mouth sores and cankers. People undergoing radiation to the head or neck will also have to deal with severe mouth or throat soreness, and many find it difficult to eat at all. I would advise anyone in this situation to consult an RD. Foods in this category are soft and smooth and low in acid, to minimize irritation. I sometimes add citrus to a dish at the end of cooking to lift its flavors. This can be left out to prevent discomfort. Most soups in the book can be blended to a smooth consistency to make eating them easier. For this I recommend using a high-speed blender, as an immersion blender will leave the food too chunky. Food should be eaten or sipped in frequent small portions and served warm instead of hot. To make foods easier to swallow, add smooth, fatty foods like avocado to, say, a smoothie and even unsalted butter to a soup.

Always take care when blending hot liquids. Fill the blender vase only halfway, and keep the lid tamped down with a cloth. This will prevent the heat from the liquid from expanding and lifting the blender lid off, which will either scald you or re-decorate your kitchen with soup.

Ann's
Tips
· ⚹ ·

NAUSEA

This category contains easy-on-the-stomach, bland-tasting, inoffensive foods and beverages: think bananas, white rice, applesauce, and plain toast.

BLAND DIET

A bland diet is made up of foods that are soft, not very spicy, and low in fat and fiber. This diet may be used to ease ulcers, heartburn, nausea, vomiting, diarrhea, and gas or may be recommended after stomach or intestinal surgery. It may also be advisable to follow a moderately bland diet leading up to or following chemotherapy infusions, particularly if you've experienced digestive side effects in the past.

HIGH FIBER

A high-fiber diet is recommended to promote regular bowel habits, manage weight, and encourage general health. This diet may be particularly important for someone who is prone to constipation or is experiencing irregularity as a result of treatment. Twenty-five to thirty-five grams of fiber per day is thought to be ideal, but increase the fiber in your diet slowly; if you're not used to it, it can cause intestinal discomfort, aka gas. As you add more dietary fiber, make sure to increase your fluid intake, too. It will help avoid constipation.

LOW FIBER

Similar to the bland diet, low-fiber diets may be necessary after stomach, gynecologic, or intestinal surgery and may be used as part of the management of treatment-induced diarrhea. Unlike the bland diet, those on a low-fiber diet can have moderate amounts of fats but need to drastically reduce fiber intake to rest bowels or intestines.

GLUTEN-FREE

Gluten is a protein found naturally in grains such as wheat, barley, rye, and triticale (a cross between wheat and rye). Gluten is also found in many processed foods to act as a binding agent. A gluten-free diet is one that excludes any gluten-containing food. Sufferers of celiac disease must avoid even trace amounts of gluten. Some others may experience a level of intolerance to this protein and feel relief by limiting intake of it. Except for some cakes and cookies, in most of the recipes where we've used the usual wheat products, you can easily substitute gluten-free breads, flours, or pastas.

NEUTROPENIC DIET

Some medical centers recommend this diet (otherwise known as "low microbial" or "low bacteria"), if neutrophil (a type of white blood cell) levels get too low to adequately protect from infection. When white blood cells are low, microbes your body typically deals with easily could send you to the ER. A neutropenic diet is low in foods that are prone to containing bacteria, helping to keep you well. Neutropenic diet restrictions vary depending on white blood cell counts, so make sure you talk to your RD for specifics. Usually raw foods, sushi, and food from buffets, salad bars, and delis are off-limits. Some medical centers also add probiotics like yogurt to this list, so it's always best to ask. These no-nos may make you feel as if you can't eat anything, but if you look through our recipes, you'll see this isn't so. There is still a lot of tasty, good food out there for you.

HEALTHY SURVIVORSHIP

A cancer survivor is defined as any person with cancer from the moment of diagnosis. Recipes in this category include foods that are beneficial for overall health and vitality. The recipes we have chosen for this category follow the American Institute of Cancer Research's rules for eating for prevention that may help to reduce the risk of recurrence. As we need to increase our fruit and vegetable intake to stay healthy, these recipes are mostly vegetable based, are low in saturated fats, have no red meats or smoked meats, and have no added sugar. That said, with the exception of sweets—which should only ever be treats—all the recipes in this book can be eaten for healthy survivorship as part of a vegetable-rich diet.

FOOD PREFERENCES

These are very basic and are to help those who followed a particular diet or lifestyle before diagnosis.

VEGAN
Recipes contain no animal products whatsoever.

VEGETARIAN
Recipes contain no meat but do include eggs and dairy.

DAIRY-FREE
Recipes without dairy. Unless also marked "vegan," these may contain animal products.

NUTS
Recipes that use either nuts or nut flours. Those who are allergic can discard where used as a garnish. Substitutes are suggested where possible.

Staples

· · · ⚜ · · ·

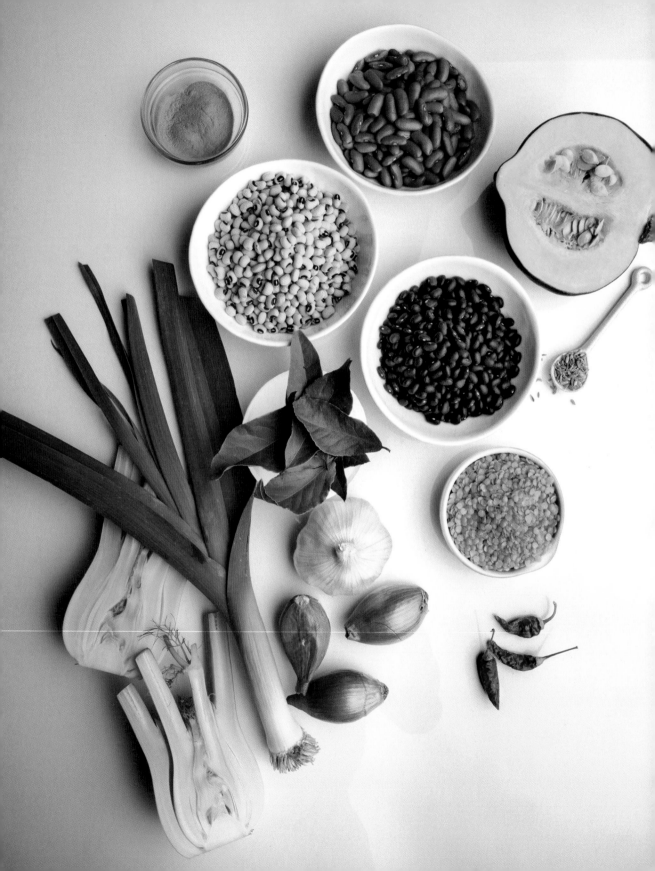

· · · · · ✳ · · · · ·

When I was going through cancer treatment, I found it important to be prepared. I always kept the basics on hand so I could cook without too much thinking or effort when the fatigue became intense. Staples are the pantry essentials and basic recipes you'll see used throughout this book. I can't do without them. They are what make cooking great food easy.

Pantry Essentials: These are the items I suggest you stock your pantry, fridge, and freezer with so you can magic up a tasty, nutritious meal without having to go to the store.

Basic Recipe Essentials: These range from instructions on how to cook basic things such as broths, beans, rice, and quinoa from scratch to how to boil an egg or prep greens for your freezer.

Speaking of the freezer, both during treatment and as a busy survivor, make your freezer your friend, your home convenience store. Use it to freeze basic home-cooked beans, greens, rice, and broths, or leftovers of a tasty soup to keep in readiness for the down times during treatment, or simply to have a good homemade meal at your fingertips that just needs defrosting if you get home late.

THE PANTRY ESSENTIALS

GROCERY BASICS

Although not listed as fridge items, it is always best to store whole-grain flours, nuts, and nut butters in the fridge to keep them fresh. The oils in them can go rancid if left on the counter. Do the same with cooking and salad oils. My bulk olive oil stays in the fridge while I decant what I need for the week into a smaller bottle that I keep on the counter.

- Almonds (sliced)
- Arborio rice
- Brown rice
- Canned beans (all kinds)
- Canned tomatoes (whole and diced only)
- Cider vinegar
- Dijon mustard
- Extra-virgin olive oil
- Lentils (French and brown)
- Maple syrup (real)
- Oats (rolled)
- Quinoa
- Raisins
- Soy sauce
- Tahini
- Walnuts (halved)
- Whole-wheat pasta
- Whole-wheat pastry flour

HERBS AND SPICES

Spice racks look nice, but they don't help your spices last. Store spices in airtight containers in a cool, dark place, like a cupboard or a drawer. I usually grind whole spices to powder as needed in a coffee grinder that I keep just for this purpose. Whole spices keep their aroma for up to a year, but ground spices generally only last about six months before the flavor fades, so if you buy ground, change them often.

- Bay leaves
- Cayenne
- Cinnamon (ground)
- Cloves (whole)
- Cumin seeds
- Curry powder (mild)
- Kosher salt
- Nutmeg (whole)
- Paprika (ground, smoked)
- Peppercorns (black)
- Rosemary (dried)
- Sea salt
- Thyme (dried)
- Turmeric (ground)

FRIDGE ITEMS

I love these items. They are multipurpose unifiers for so many recipes that make meals in their own right. Maybe not the butter or the coconut oil, but the rest all easily lend themselves to quick and delicious dishes.

- Butter (unsalted; pastured, if available)
- Coconut oil
- Eggs (hormone- and antibiotic-free)
- Feta cheese
- Miso (white)
- Parmesan cheese (chunk)
- Plain Greek yogurt (whole milk or 2%)
- Tofu

FREEZER ITEMS

With these in your freezer, a meal with the taste and high-nutrition value of fresh fruits and vegetables is always at hand—without all the prep. Don't defrost them before using. The nutrients tend to leach out as they soften.

- Baby lima beans
- Blueberries
- Garden peas
- Green or French beans
- Kale (or collards)
- Leaf spinach
- Mixed berries

FRESH PRODUCE

Last but not least, the produce you should always have on hand. These are the aromatics—onions, garlic, and shallots that, along with carrots and celery, make the flavor base for so many soups and stews—while lemons, gingerroot, and parsley add delicious accents. I've added beets to this list because I love them, and, when vacuum-packed, they are particularly trouble-free. Apples and bananas are great year-round fruits that can be used for simple desserts and smoothies. Store onions, garlic, and shallots on the countertop—bananas, too. Everything else can stay in the fridge.

- Apples
- Bananas
- Beets (vacuum-packed)
- Carrots
- Celery
- Garlic
- Gingerroot
- Lemons
- Onions
- Parsley (flat-leaf)
- Shallots

THE BASIC RECIPE ESSENTIALS

Broths and beans are the building blocks of good food and essential elements of a vegetable-based diet. Although you may not feel like making these recipes during treatment, they're worth it. They will help you to make quick nourishing meals straight from your freezer.

Basic Vegetable Broth

Vegetable stock is really easy to make and stores perfectly in the freezer. This recipe is a classic and uses whole vegetables, but you can also mix together the peelings from carrots, potatoes, and onions or leek tops, kale ribs, or parsley stalks to make stock. Add a bay leaf and some peppercorns and you're on your way.

Meal: Basics

Main Ingredients: Water, soup vegetables

Prep Time: 20 minutes

Cook Time: 60 minutes

MAKES APPROXIMATELY 5 QUARTS

2 large yellow onions, unpeeled, cut in half

2 whole cloves

3 leeks, trimmed and washed well, dark tops reserved

8 cloves garlic, smashed but not peeled

4 large carrots, scrubbed and cut into 3 equal lengths, then cut in half lengthwise

2 waxy potatoes, scrubbed and quartered

2 stalks celery, scrubbed and each cut into 3 pieces

1 bay leaf

2 sprigs Italian parsley

½ teaspoon black peppercorns

5 quarts water

Sea salt, to taste

1. Stud the onions with the cloves. Cut the white part of the trimmed leeks into three equal lengths, then in half lengthwise. Set aside. Cut the tender parts of the dark leek tops into 3-inch lengths.

2. In a 7-quart pot, cover the onions, leeks, garlic, carrots, potatoes, celery, bay leaf, parsley, and black peppercorns with enough water to completely cover the vegetables by 1 inch or so.

3. Bring to a boil over high heat. Cover the pot and reduce the heat to low. Gently simmer the vegetables for 1 hour.

4. Taste for salt and adjust the seasonings. Strain the stock and let cool. Discard the vegetables. Use immediately or bag and freeze.

Ann's Tips

· 🍴 ·

You can make this broth in a slow cooker overnight by placing all the ingredients into the cooker and cooking on low for 10 hours, or on high for 5 hours.

If you make broth with vegetable peelings, go easy on using too many from pungent vegetables such as celery root (celeriac), unless you want your broth to taste only of them, that is.

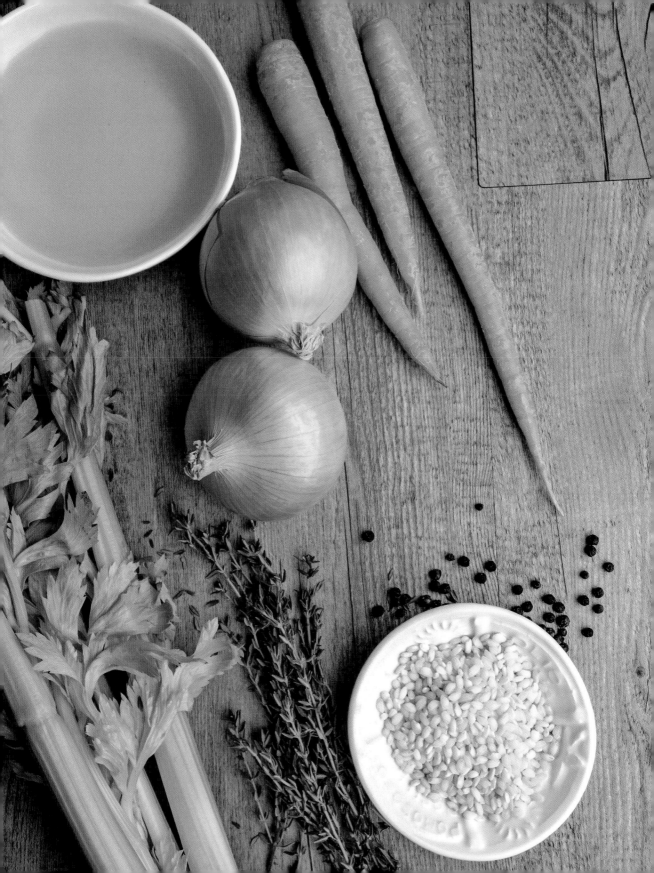

Quick, Rich Chicken Broth

Meal: Basics

Main Ingredient: Chicken

Prep Time: 15 minutes

Cook Time: 45 to 60 minutes

MAKES 10 TO 12 CUPS

Broths are soothing and nutritious. This one is really quick and easy to make and is quite delicious. You can make it in an hour on the stove top, but if you have a slow cooker, just put in all the ingredients and let it cook all day (or night). Either way, you will have a rich-tasting chicken broth to use as a base for some of the simple, nourishing soups in this book.

6 (antibiotic-free) skinless, bone-in chicken thighs

1 medium carrot, scrubbed and halved

1 stalk celery, scrubbed and halved

1 bay leaf

1 teaspoon black peppercorns

1 medium onion, peeled and halved

4 whole cloves

1 teaspoon sea salt, plus more to taste

1. In a large stockpot, place the chicken thighs, carrot, celery, bay leaf, and pepper-corns. Stud each onion half with 2 cloves and add to the pot. Sprinkle with 1 teaspoon sea salt.
2. Add enough cold water to cover the chicken and vegetables by 1 inch. Bring to a boil. Cover and reduce the heat to medium-low. Cook for 45 minutes. Taste for salt. If you want to eat the chicken, remove it now. Otherwise let it cook 15 to 20 minutes longer for an even more flavorful broth.

Ann's Tips

· ✳ ·

If you remove the chicken from the broth after 45 minutes, carve the meat from the bones, return the bones to the broth, and cook for 20 to 30 minutes more.

Basic Poached Fish

This method and broth will work for all kinds of fish, including salmon. When buying fillets of any large fish, always insist on having the thick piece from behind the head, and not the thin, pointed tail end. This will ensure a uniform thickness of fish for an even cooking time.

Meal: Main

Main Ingredient: Seafood

Prep Time: 15 minutes

Cook Time: 20 minutes

SERVES 4 TO 6

1 large shallot, peeled

2 whole cloves

2 cloves garlic, peeled and smashed

1 small carrot, scrubbed and halved lengthwise

½ fennel bulb, cut into ¼-inch slices, stalks and fronds removed

1 bay leaf

½ teaspoon whole peppercorns (optional)

½ teaspoon sea salt, or to taste

2 quarts water

1 to 1½ pounds fish fillets (cod, hake, Chilean sea bass, or salmon) either in one thick piece or cut into 3-inch slices

1. Make the broth: Stud the shallot with the cloves. In a sauté pan, add the shallot, garlic, carrot, fennel, bay leaf, and peppercorns, if using. Stir in ½ teaspoon of salt and cover with cold water. Bring to a boil over medium-high heat. As soon as the water starts to bubble, cover, reduce the heat to low, and simmer for 10 minutes, or until the vegetables are soft. Taste for salt.

2. Add the fish fillets to the pan, in a single layer if sliced. Add extra hot water to just cover the fish if needed. Increase heat to medium and bring to a simmer. As soon as the water starts to bubble, reduce heat to low, cover, and cook the fish at a bare simmer for 10 minutes.

3. After 10 minutes, if the fillets are in one piece, turn the heat off and leave the fish to steam in the broth for another 5 minutes. If the fillets are in slices, remove the fish with a spatula and transfer to a plate. Discard the broth and vegetables. Serve the fish with your chosen sauce.

Ann's Tips

· ✲ ·

If you are poaching a piece of salmon fillet to eat cold, after you've brought the broth back to a boil in step 2, cover the pan tightly, turn off the flame, and leave the salmon to poach in the broth as it cools, about 30 minutes. The fish will be perfectly cooked.

Quick Tomato Sauce

This is the sauce base I use for nearly all the tomato pasta dishes we eat at home. It is the easiest thing you could ever make, and quick, too. It freezes like a dream, so you can always have it on hand for a fast dinner.

2 tablespoons extra-virgin olive oil

1 to 2 cloves garlic, peeled and sliced thin lengthwise

1 small dried red pepper (optional), seeds removed

1 (28-ounce) can chopped tomatoes

Sea salt, to taste

Meal: Basics, Sauces

Main Ingredient: Tomatoes

Prep Time: 10 minutes

Cook Time: 15 minutes

MAKES ABOUT 1½ CUPS SAUCE

1. Heat the oil in a sauté pan over medium-high heat. When the oil starts to shimmer, add the garlic and stir-fry until it just begins to turn golden, about 1 minute. If you want a spicy sauce, add the pepper.

2. Add the tomatoes and a pinch of salt. There will be a lot of spitting and hissing as the tomatoes hit the hot oil. Reduce the heat to medium-low and continue to cook the tomatoes down until most of the juices have evaporated and the tomatoes have taken on a more orangey hue, about 10 minutes. If the sauce looks like it's drying out too much, add a little water. Taste for seasoning. Freeze if not using immediately.

In the summertime, when tomatoes are at their peak, use 2 pounds of ripe Roma or beefsteak tomatoes in place of the canned tomatoes.

Ann's Tips

· 🕊 ·

Basic Vinaigrette

Meal: Basics, Sauces

Main Ingredients:
Extra-virgin olive oil,
White wine vinegar

Prep Time: 5 minutes

Cook Time: 0 minutes

MAKES ¼ CUP

An oil-to-vinegar ratio of three-to-one (3:1) is the key to this basic 101 vinaigrette salad dressing; it is the dressing from which all others start. You can change the vinegar you use, add citrus, flavor it with chopped herbs, you name it. Get comfortable with this, and you can make any dressing.

1 tablespoon white wine vinegar

Sea salt and freshly ground black pepper, to taste

Pinch of brown sugar or honey (optional)

3 tablespoons extra-virgin olive oil

1 tablespoon water, or to taste

1. In a bowl, whisk together the vinegar, salt, pepper, and sugar, if using, until the salt has dissolved.
2. Gradually beat in the olive oil until well blended. Taste for seasoning. If the vinegar is too strong, add some water a little at a time.

Ann's Tips

· ⚶ ·

For a lighter dressing, substitute 1 tablespoon of water for one of the tablespoons of olive oil.

Although my mother taught me to add a pinch of sugar to this dressing, I no longer do so. If I want a little sweetness, I add some diced apple or a tablespoonful of raisins instead.

Soft- and Hard-Boiled Eggs

Hard-boiled eggs are your safest egg option during treatment and make an easy, nutritious snack eaten straight from the fridge.

4 large eggs (antibiotic-free)

Pinch of sea salt

Meal: Basics, Breakfast

Main Ingredient: Eggs

Cook Time: 7½ to 10 minutes

SERVES 4

1. Gently place the eggs in a medium saucepan and cover them with cold water. Add a pinch of salt. The salt will set any seeping egg white, should an egg crack during boiling.
2. Bring the water to a rolling boil over medium-high heat, about 5 minutes. Cover, turn the heat down to medium, and cook for 2½ minutes for soft-boiled eggs or 5 minutes for hard-boiled eggs.
3. Remove the pan from the heat and place it in the sink. Run cold water over the eggs until the water in the pan is cold. Peel if eating immediately. If not eating warm, leave the eggs to sit in the cold water until completely cooled. Store in the fridge to use as needed. They will keep for 3 to 4 days.

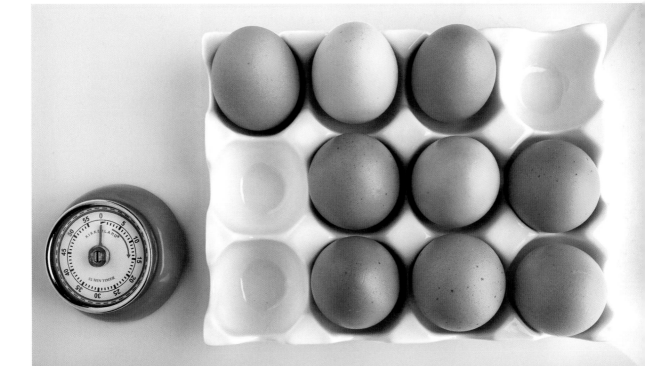

Poached Eggs

Meal: Basics, breakfast, lunch

Main Ingredient: Eggs

Prep Time: 0 minutes

Cook Time: 5 minutes

Poaching is a great low-fat way to prepare eggs. Very fresh eggs work best for poaching. Their firm, domed whites will make them easier to handle. If you are in treatment, particularly if you are on a neutropenic diet, it's best to cook the eggs until the yolks are hard and completely cooked through.

4 large eggs (antibiotic-free)

Water

1 teaspoon apple cider vinegar or white wine vinegar

Pinch of sea salt

1. Add about a 1-inch depth of hot water to a frying pan. Add the teaspoon of vinegar and a pinch of salt. Heat over high heat until the water just starts to boil. Reduce the heat to low. The water should be barely moving.
2. Carefully break the eggs into the water—the whites will start to set immediately. Cover with a lid and cook, occasionally spooning water over the eggs, until the whites have set and the yolks are cooked to your liking and have an opaque film over them, 3 to 5 minutes. If you need to be sure the yolks are hard, cook the eggs for 7 minutes to be on the safe side.

Basic Brown Rice

This is the simplest way to make al dente brown rice. This method of cooking uses little water and a lot of steam. It is pretty much foolproof if you have a pot with a tight-fitting lid. The secret is to stop yourself from peeking—from the moment the rice starts to boil until the steaming period is over.

2 cups long-grain brown rice, washed in several changes of water

2⅓ cups water or stock

Sea salt, to taste

1. Place the rice in a heavy pot with a tight-fitting lid. Add the water and salt. Bring to a boil. Cover the pot and turn the heat down to low.
2. Simmer the rice gently for 40 minutes. Turn the heat off and leave the rice to steam for 10 to 15 minutes with the lid on. Fluff with a fork and serve. Freeze flat in 1-quart freezer bags if not eating immediately.

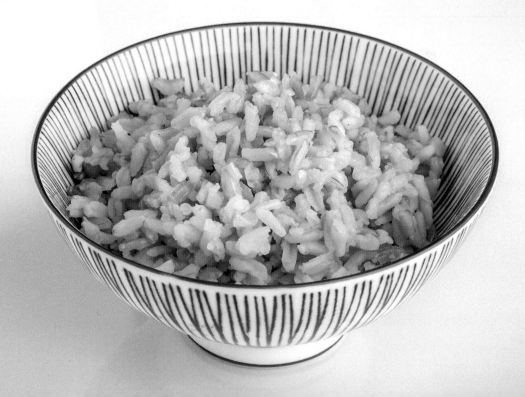

White Rice

Meal: Basics

Main Ingredient: White long-grain rice

Prep Time: 5 minutes

Cook Time: 20 minutes, plus 10 minutes resting time

MAKES APPROXIMATELY 4 CUPS

It may seem counterintuitive, but despite the benefits of whole grains, there are times when it's actually better for you to eat white rice. When your stomach is upset through chemo or if you've undergone abdominal surgery or your intestines are irritated, foods rich in fiber can be difficult to digest. This is when your doctor may recommend you eat a bland diet. A bland diet consists of poached chicken or fish, steamed vegetables, and white rice, with no raw foods or whole grains. In these circumstances, you'll find white rice to be a boon. It is a quick source of energy and it's easy to digest. My favorite choice is super-long-grain basmati rice. Not only is it slightly lower on the glycemic index than other white rice (according to the American Diabetic Association), it has a distinctive and deliciously aromatic flavor. When you're feeling better, it's great as an occasional accompaniment to a tasty curry or stir-fry.

2 cups long-grain white rice

3 cups water or stock

Sea salt, to taste

1. Place the rice, water, and salt in a heavy pot with a tight-fitting lid. Bring to a rolling boil. Cover the pot and reduce the heat to low. Simmer the rice gently for 20 minutes. Do not lift the lid.
2. Turn the heat off. Keep the rice covered and leave the rice to steam for 10 to 15 minutes. No peeking!
3. Fluff with a fork and serve. Freeze flat in 1-quart freezer bags if not eating immediately.

Basic Quinoa

Quinoa is a great grain that has complete protein. As quick cooking as white rice, quinoa can stand in for brown rice or whole-wheat couscous. It has a bitter coating that needs to be rinsed off, but these days it is often sold prewashed, so omit step 1 if it is.

2 cups white, red, or black quinoa

1½ cups water or broth

½ teaspoon sea salt

Meal: Basics

Main Ingredient: Quinoa

Prep Time: 5 minutes

Cook Time: 20 minutes

MAKES ABOUT 5 CUPS

1. In a fine sieve, rinse the quinoa a few times. Drain well.
2. In a heavy pot, bring the washed quinoa and water to a boil with a pinch of salt. Cover, reduce the heat to let simmer, and cook for 20 minutes or until the spiral around the quinoa seed has come loose and the quinoa is tender but still chewy. If there is any remaining water, drain it off. Use immediately or cool and store in the refrigerator or freezer.

Ann's Tips

For more flavor, try adding a clove of garlic, a scallion, or a sprig of rosemary or cilantro to the water while the quinoa is cooking.

Mashed Potatoes
with Nutmeg

Meal: Sides

Main Ingredient:
Potato, Butter

Prep Time: 10 minutes

Cook Time: 15 minutes

SERVES 4 TO 6

I love mashed potatoes. They are the most comforting food I know of. I've used unsalted pastured butter in mashed potatoes, and to me it is delicious and soothing and turns the humble potato into a real treat. Eating potatoes mashed with nutmeg takes me back to my mom's kitchen and the taste of motherly love. Pure comfort and joy.

1½ pounds Yukon Gold, Idaho, or russet potatoes, peeled and quartered

2 teaspoons sea salt, plus more to taste

2 tablespoons unsalted pasture-raised butter (see Ann's Tips, next page)

½ teaspoon freshly ground nutmeg, or to taste

1. Put the potatoes into a stockpot or other large pot. Cover with cold water by 1 inch. Add 2 teaspoons of salt and bring to a boil. Partially cover and simmer until very tender, about 15 minutes, depending on the size of the potatoes. Reserve 1 cup of cooking water and drain the potatoes.

2. Return the drained potatoes to the pot and, using a potato masher or fork, mash the potatoes with the butter and 1 tablespoon of their cooking water or with as much is needed to reach your preferred consistency. Sprinkle the nutmeg over the potatoes and mash it in. Taste for salt. Eat.

For higher fiber, cook and mash the potatoes with their skins on.

Use pasture-raised butter like Organic Valley brand, if you can get it. Dairy products, such as butter, from pastured animals have better nutritional profiles, being higher in conjugated linoleic acids (CLA) than regular butter. (It is still high in saturated fat, however.)

If you'd rather not use butter at all, use either 2 tablespoons olive oil or ¼ cup plain Greek yogurt with the freshly grated nutmeg.

Ann's
Tips
· ✶ ·

Steaming and Freezing Greens at Home

Meal: Basics

Main Ingredient: Leafy greens

Prep Time: 15 minutes

Cook Time: 5 minutes

SERVES 3 TO 4

Greens cooked this way are ready to be quickly sautéed in olive oil, garlic, and some dried chili (if you like spicy), or frozen and stored for another use. It may seem as if there won't be enough water to cook them in, but there will be, especially once the kale has given up its own moisture.

1 bunch curly or lacinato (dinosaur) kale, collards, chard, or spinach

Sea salt, to taste

1. Strip out the tough stems and discard (see Ann's Tips, below).
2. Wash the greens in a sink full of cold water. Transfer the greens to a large pot with the water that clings to their leaves.
3. Set the pot of wet kale over high heat. Sprinkle the kale with a little salt and cover. The water on the leaves will make its way to the bottom of the pan and start to steam and wilt the greens. Cook until the kale is completely wilted and reduced in volume, about 5 minutes, turning the leaves once for even cooking.
4. Drain into a colander and set under cold running water to stop the cooking. Squeeze out any excess moisture and roughly chop. Fluff the chopped kale, bag, and freeze for further use.

Ann's Tips

If you use this method for collards or other tougher-leaved greens, add ½ cup of water, but not more.

Spinach and chard are very soft and will wilt after 1 to 2 minutes.

The stems of chard are edible, but they take longer to cook than the leaves. Reserve for another use, or sauté until just soft, then add the leaves.

Spicy Chickpeas in Chipotle Broth

This recipe makes delicious chickpeas with a nutritious, spicy broth you can add to soups and stews. These chickpeas freeze well, too, and are a tasty alternative to canned.

2 cups dried chickpeas

1 bay leaf

3 cloves garlic, peeled

1 dried chipotle pepper

1 tablespoon extra-virgin olive oil

Sea salt, to taste

Meal: Basics

Main Ingredient:
Chickpeas (garbanzos)

Prep Time: 10 hours, plus 6 to 8 hours for soaking

Cook Time: 90 to 120 minutes

MAKES APPROXIMATELY 8 CUPS

1. Rinse the dried chickpeas and put them into a large bowl. Add 4 times their volume of water and cover with a cloth. Leave to soak for 6 to 8 hours or overnight.
2. Drain the chickpeas and put them into a pot. Add just enough water to cover completely. Bring to a boil, removing with a slotted spoon any scum that forms.
3. Add the bay leaf, garlic, and dried chipotle. Drizzle with the olive oil. Lower the heat, cover, and simmer gently until they are tender but not mushy, 1½ to 2 hours. Cooking time will depend on the age of the chickpeas. Add salt to taste.
4. Use as needed. Bag and freeze any extra for another dish.

If you have a slow cooker, use it for these chickpeas. You don't even need to soak them—just add enough water to cover the chickpeas by 2 inches. Everything else stays the same except for the cooking time, which should be 6 to 8 hours, either all night or all day.

Ann's Tips

· ✲ ·

Basic Beans #1

Meal: Basics

Main Ingredient: Black beans

Prep Time: 10 hours, plus 6 to 8 hours for soaking

Cook Time: 40 to 60 minutes

MAKES APPROXIMATELY 8 CUPS

This recipe is good for black, red kidney, and pinto beans and black-eyed peas. There are also instructions to make them in a slow cooker. If you are adding them to soups or stews, the broth they make is delicious.

1 cup dried beans

4 cups water

2 small shallots, peeled

1 bay leaf

3 sprigs cilantro, stem and leaves, washed well (optional for black beans)

1 teaspoon extra-virgin olive oil

½ teaspoon sea salt, or to taste

1. Rinse the beans under the tap. Put them into a bowl large enough to hold them and the water. Cover with a plate or plastic wrap and leave to soak for 6 to 8 hours or overnight. They should double in size.

2. Drain the soaked beans, rinse them, and put them into a heavy pot with the shallots, bay leaf, and cilantro, if using. Add enough water just to cover the beans, and add the olive oil.

3. Bring the beans to a boil. With a slotted spoon, remove any scum that forms. Boil for 10 minutes, cover, and reduce the heat to low. Simmer until the beans still hold their shape but are tender, 40 minutes to 1 hour depending on the age of the beans.

4. Remove the cilantro, shallots, and bay leaf. Add the sea salt. Use the beans or store them in the fridge or freezer.

SLOW COOKER

You don't need to soak the beans for this. Rinse them and put them in a slow cooker together with the shallots, bay leaf, and cilantro, if using. Add enough water to cover the beans by a good 2 inches. Leave to cook for 6 to 8 hours. Add salt when the beans are cooked.

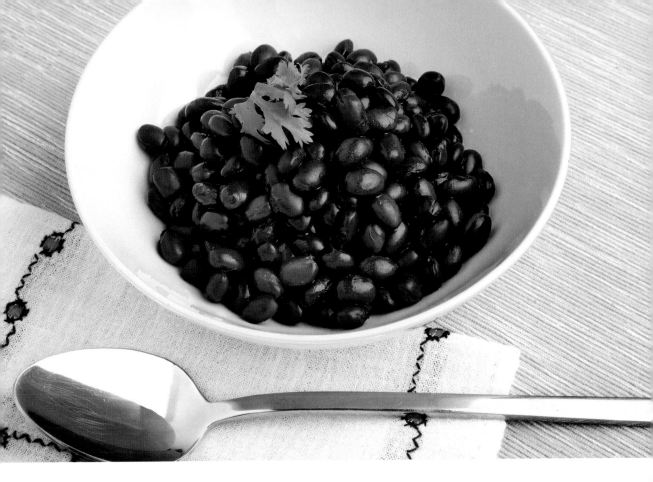

These beans are great to use in soups and stews instead of canned. If you didn't remember to soak them overnight, use this quick method instead of step 1 on page 38:

1. Put the beans into a large saucepan. Add 8 cups of water and bring to a rolling boil. Cover and cook for 1 minute to build up steam.
2. Turn the heat off and leave the beans covered and untouched for 1 hour to soften.
3. Proceed with step 2.

Basic Beans #2

Meal: Basics

Main Ingredient: White beans

Prep Time: 6 to 8 hours for soaking

Cook Time: 20 to 30 minutes

MAKES APPROXIMATELY 8 CUPS

This is a basic recipe for cooking all dried white beans: cannellini, Great Northern, navy, lima, or broad beans. Dried beans will not soften if cooked in salted water. Do not add any salt or stock until the beans are soft. The garlic, oil, and herbs will give them plenty of flavor. The broth they cook in is delicious and is a great addition to soups and stews.

1 cup dried white beans

1 small sprig rosemary

3 cloves garlic, peeled and smashed

Extra-virgin olive oil

1. Soak the beans: Rinse the dried beans in water and put them in a large bowl. Cover with at least 4 times their volume of water, cover with plastic wrap, and let sit in a cool place overnight.
2. Drain and rinse the beans and put them into a pot with a heavy lid. Add just enough cold water to cover them.
3. Add the rosemary, garlic, and a drizzle of olive oil. Bring the beans to a boil. Cover, reduce the heat, and simmer them gently for 20 to 30 minutes or until the beans are tender but not mushy. The cooking time will depend on the size and age of the beans. Smaller and newer beans will require a shorter cooking time, so check on them after 20 minutes.
4. Use the beans or store them in the fridge or freezer.

SLOW COOKER

You don't need to soak the beans for this. Rinse them and put them in a slow cooker together with the garlic, rosemary, and olive oil. Add enough water to cover the beans by a good 2 inches. Leave to cook for 6 to 8 hours. Add salt when the beans are cooked.

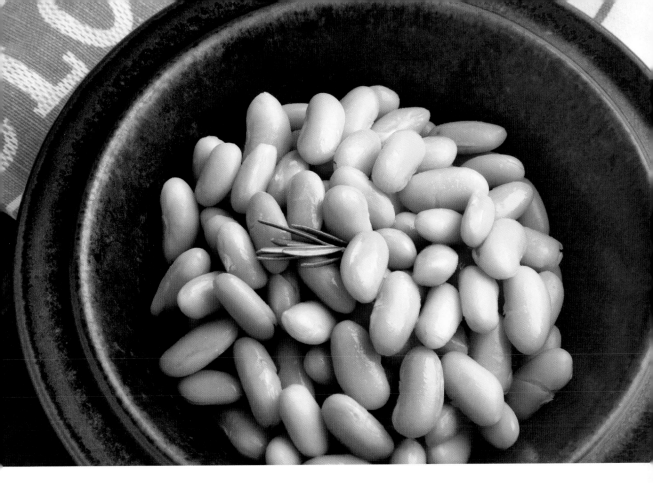

These beans are great to use in soups and stews instead of canned. If you didn't remember to soak them overnight, use this quick method instead of step 1 on page 40:

page 40

1. Put the beans into a large saucepan. Add 8 cups of water and bring to a rolling boil. Cover and cook for 1 minute to build up steam.
2. Turn the heat off and leave the beans covered and untouched for 1 hour to soften.
3. Proceed with step 2.

Ann's
Tips
· ⚹ ·

Simple

· · · ✈ · · ·

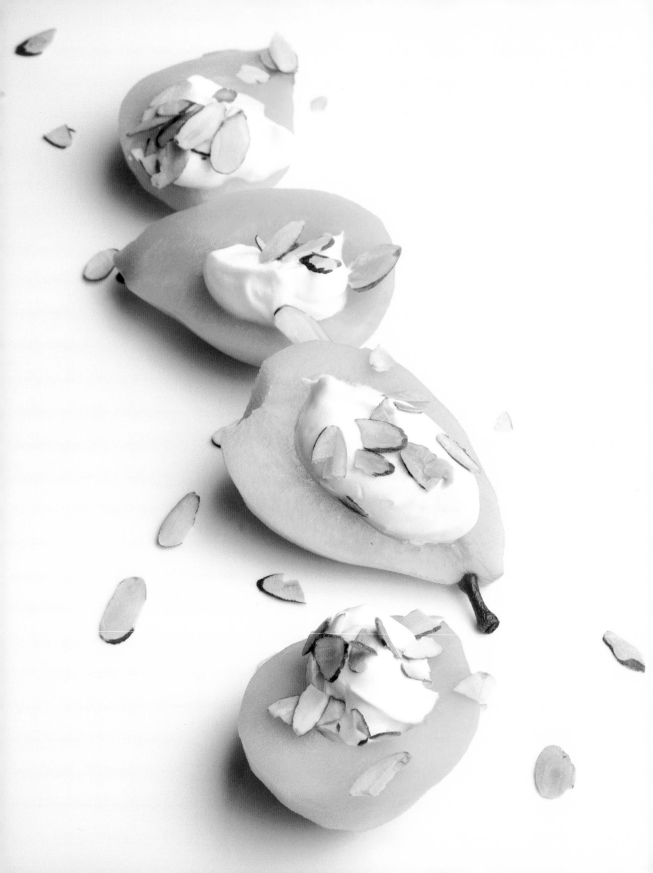

S imple food is delicious food, and it's lucky for us that it is. Cancer treatment causes terrible fatigue. It doesn't matter whether you're going through chemo, radiation, or hormone therapy—fatigue comes with the territory. When I went through treatment for my second cancer, the crushing tiredness that came after each chemo infusion meant that cooking became either defrosting and heating up some soup or other meal that I'd made ahead of time just to cope with this miserable moment, or reaching for tasty recipes that weren't too energy intensive, simple foods I could nourish myself with before flopping back on the couch. Then came radiation, with its cumulative fatigue. By the end of six weeks, I, who am usually a night bird, was barely able to stay awake to make dinner.

Happily, it turns out that some of the tastiest things we can eat are among the fastest, easiest meals to throw together. To save time and energy, I've purposely kept the prep in the following recipes to 15 to 20 minutes, each with four or five fresh items to put to the knife. The other ingredients are pantry items like dried herbs or spices or canned beans, items that require no more effort than opening a jar or a can and adding a pinch here or a cup there. Frozen fruits and veggies are also a great standby when speed and simplicity are what's needed. I find frozen peas, leaf spinach, and blueberries to be keepers (see the Stock Your Pantry sidebar on page 46). If your local supermarket offers precut veggies, go for it. They save time and valuable energy. After all, this isn't cooking boot camp; these are just easy solutions to help you look after yourself through the worst of your treatment, deliciously and simply.

STOCK YOUR PANTRY

It's easier to keep things simple if your pantry is stocked with basics. Make sure to always have dried and canned goods such as rice, pasta, canned beans, and canned tomatoes on hand, and keep some of your favorite frozen vegetables ready in the freezer, too, like frozen peas, edamame, or baby lima beans for a quick protein add-in, and whole-leaf spinach or kale for a fast infusion of greens. Basic herbs and spices are a big help. You won't need every one, but if you have bay leaves, rosemary, thyme, oregano, cumin, cayenne, and curry powder, you can make almost anything. See the full list of pantry basics to have on hand on page 18.

PLAN AHEAD

Many soups and one-pot meals can be made ahead of time and frozen in single or double portions so that on your worst days all you have to do is defrost and nuke them. Use the "bag and freeze" technique to make this easier.

BAG AND FREEZE: FOR 1–2 PORTIONS:

1. Write the name and the date of the food you wish to freeze on a 1-quart ziplock bag. Add the portion you'd like to freeze. Leave plenty of room at the top so you can close it without overflow, and so that it will be relatively flat when sealed and on its side.
2. Before sealing the bag, smooth together the empty top sides to push out any remaining air. Close the zip. You can open a corner slightly to push out any existing air, then reseal tightly.
3. Lay the bag flat in the bottom of the freezer. It will freeze into a stackable flat block, allowing you to freeze several bags together one on top of the other.

FATIGUE

Research has shown that gentle exercise is one of the best antidotes to fatigue. So even if you don't feel much like it, get up and take a walk around the block. Afterward, it won't be so hard to make yourself some dinner.

Breakfast Quinoa with Green Tea and Dates

Meal: Breakfast

Main Ingredient: Quinoa

Prep Time: 10 minutes

Cook Time: 15 minutes

SERVES 4

HEALTH CONSIDERATIONS: GLUTEN-FREE; IN TREATMENT; EASY TO SWALLOW; NAUSEA; FATIGUE; NEUTROPENIC DIET

FOOD PREFERENCE: VEGAN; VEGETARIAN; NUTS

This tasty vegan breakfast treat is quick to make and deliciously easy to eat no matter where you are in treatment. It uses the Japanese tradition of steeping cooked grains in green tea and flavorings to make a simple meal, except here it's not the usual rice but quinoa. Thanks to the addition of chopped dates, this quick porridge is naturally sweet, and toasted nuts add a healthy crunch. It really does make for a great start to the day.

> ## Health Tip
> While green tea is naturally caffeinated, it contains an amino acid called L-theanine, which helps to promote a sense of calm.

2 cups cooked quinoa (Basic Quinoa, page 33)

2 cups brewed green tea (sencha)

⅓ cup coarsely chopped dates

Pinch of sea salt

⅓ cups dry-toasted sliced almonds (see Ann's Tips, next page)

1 cup diced summer fruit and/or berries

Plain Greek yogurt or milk of your choice (optional)

1. Combine the quinoa, tea, and dates in a saucepan and bring to a boil over high heat, about 3 minutes. Add a pinch of salt and reduce the heat to medium-low.

Cover and simmer, until the tea is absorbed, about 10 minutes, stirring from time to time toward the end of cooking.

2. Stir in the almonds. Serve immediately with berries and diced fruit. Add a dollop of Greek yogurt or a drizzle of milk, if desired.

Ann's Tips

· ✦ ·

Dry-toasting is easy. Take a small, heavy skillet (cast-iron is best, if you have one) and heat the skillet briefly over medium heat, then add the nuts. You don't need any oil—all nuts have enough on their own. Toast the nuts, shaking the pan until they have just started to turn golden. Turn off the heat and immediately tip the nuts into a bowl. If you leave them to cool in the pan, they will continue to cook on its hot surface and can burn.

If your mouth is sore, you may want to skip the nuts.

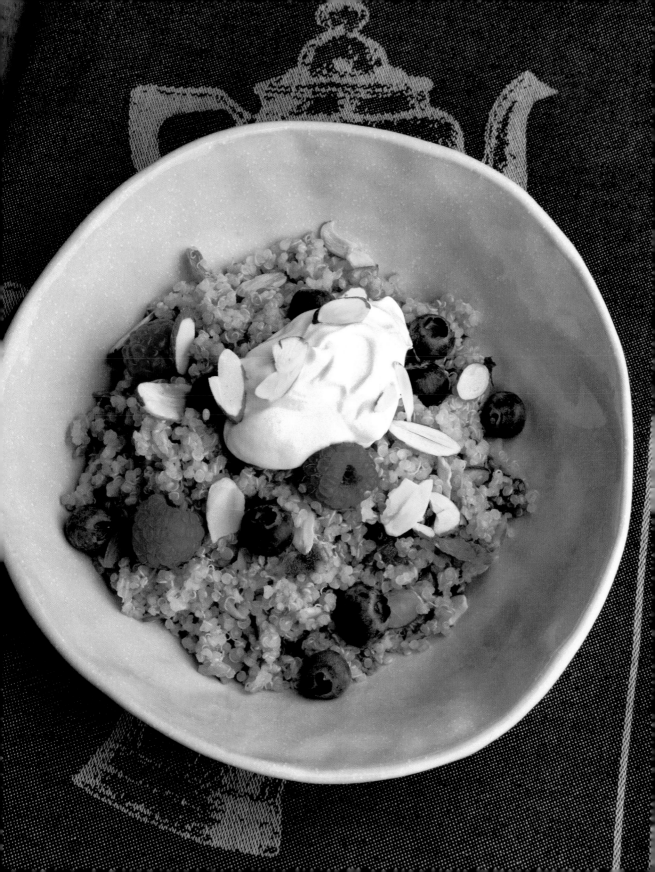

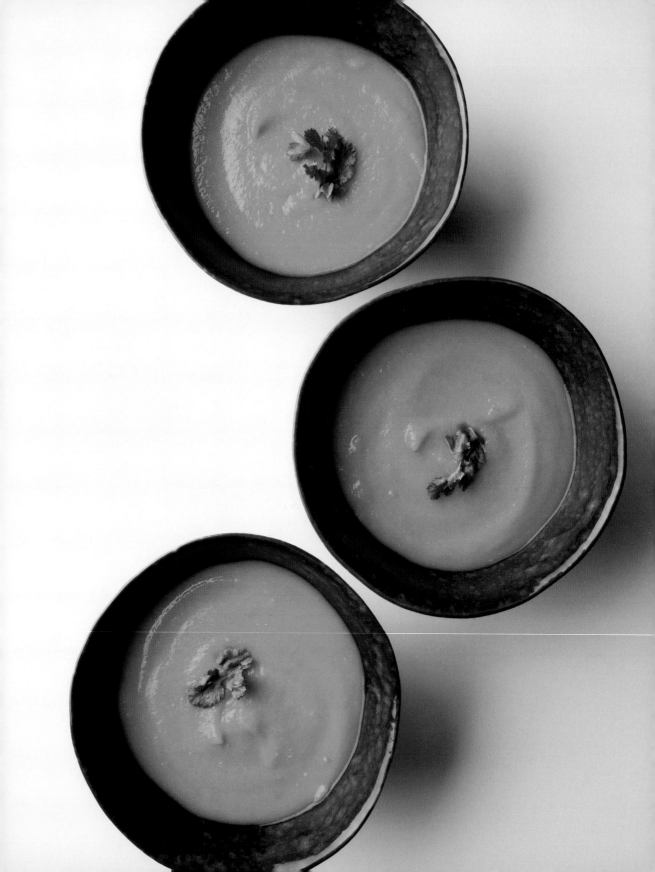

Sweet Potato and Tomato Soup

HEALTH CONSIDERATIONS: IN TREATMENT; GLUTEN-FREE; NEUTROPENIC DIET; HEALTHY SURVIVORSHIP

FOOD PREFERENCE: DAIRY-FREE; VEGAN; VEGETARIAN

Meal: Main, Soup

Main Ingredients: Sweet potatoes, Tomatoes

Prep Time: 20 minutes

Cook Time: 40 minutes

SERVES 4 TO 6

My friend Gaye Sandler first made this soup for me when I was getting over my kidney surgery. It is simplicity itself. There's very little chopping with this quick, easy, and delicious soup and it's almost foolproof. Studies have shown that the lycopene in tomatoes becomes more accessible through cooking, plus sweet potatoes contain vitamins A, C, and B_6. Who knew eating your ABCs could be so enjoyable!

2 tablespoons extra-virgin olive oil

1 large Spanish onion, diced

1 dried red chili, seeds removed (optional)

1 bay leaf

1½ pounds sweet potatoes, peeled and cut into ½-inch cubes

1 to 2 teaspoons maple syrup (optional)

1 (28-ounce) can diced tomatoes

4 cups Basic Vegetable Broth (page 21) or water

Sea salt and freshly ground black pepper, to taste

Greek yogurt, for garnish (optional)

2 tablespoons chopped cilantro, for garnish (optional)

1. Heat the oil over medium-high heat. Add the onion, chili, bay leaf, and sweet potatoes and sauté for 2 minutes. Reduce the heat to medium and cook, stirring occasionally, for 10 to 15 minutes, or until both the onion and sweet potatoes are slightly caramelized and golden.

2. Raise the heat to medium-high. Add the maple syrup, if using. Stir to mix and sauté for 30 seconds to 1 minute. Add the tomatoes and cook, 5 to 7 minutes, or until the tomatoes have turned orangey-red. Add the broth and sprinkle with salt. Stir well and bring to a slow boil. Reduce the heat to medium-low and

simmer for another 20 minutes, or until the potatoes can be smashed against the sides of the pan.

3. Remove the bay leaf and puree using an immersion blender, or puree small bits in batches in an upright blender. If the soup seems too thick for your taste, add a little extra broth to achieve the desired consistency. Taste for seasonings and adjust if needed. Return the soup to the pot and reheat gently. If you are on a neutropenic diet, add the chopped cilantro and cook for a few minutes.

4. To serve, sprinkle each bowl with 2 teaspoons of the chopped cilantro (if it hasn't been added yet), a grind or two of black pepper, and a dollop of Greek yogurt, if desired.

Ann's Tips

· ⊤ ·

Always keep canned, unseasoned diced or whole tomatoes in your pantry. They are one of the most useful ingredients in home cooking and are always a good choice for soups and sauces in the winter months when fresh tomatoes are anemic looking and tasteless. Go for tomatoes in BPA-free cans, like Muir Glen organic brand, or the Italian Pomi brand Tetra-paks.

If you are a meat eater, this can be also be made with Quick, Rich Chicken Broth (page 24).

Vegan Caldo Verde

HEALTH CONSIDERATIONS: GLUTEN-FREE; IN TREATMENT; HIGH FIBER; EASY TO SWALLOW; HEALTHY SURVIVORSHIP; NAUSEA

FOOD PREFERENCE: DAIRY-FREE; VEGAN; VEGETARIAN

Meal: Main

Main Ingredient: Kale, Potatoes

Prep Time: 20 minutes

Cook Time: 30 minutes

SERVES 4 TO 6

This simple, smoky-tasting vegan soup is a great way to eat kale. I prefer to use lacinato kale, but the soup will taste just as good with any variety your store has, including bagged baby kale. Caldo verde is traditionally made with chorizo sausage, but I've used smoked paprika instead. Smoked paprika is a great addition to your pantry. It naturally gives food a smoky flavor and meatiness that usually only come with the addition of smoked bacon or ham bones, which unfortunately are not part of a healthy diet. This soup proves you don't have to give up on taste if you give up what might have once seemed like essential ingredients.

2 tablespoons extra-virgin olive oil, plus extra for drizzling

2 cloves garlic, minced

2 teaspoons dried rosemary, or 1 small sprig fresh rosemary, leaves stripped and chopped

1 medium onion, diced

2 large Yukon Gold potatoes, unpeeled, washed, and cut into 1-inch dice

2½ teaspoons sea salt, or to taste

1 teaspoon smoked paprika

6 cups water or Basic Vegetable Broth (page 21)

Freshly ground black pepper, to taste

1 (1-pound) bag baby kale (see Ann's Tips, next page)

3 or 4 sprigs flat-leaf parsley, leaves stripped and coarsely chopped

1. Heat the olive oil in a 5-quart Dutch oven over medium-high heat. Add the garlic and rosemary. Cook until the garlic just begins to color, about 2 minutes. Add the onion and cook until it starts to become translucent. Add the potatoes and cook, stirring, for 1 minute. Sprinkle with salt, cover, reduce the heat to

medium, and let the vegetables cook for 5 to 8 minutes, stirring from time to time to prevent sticking. The onion should be soft, and the potatoes a little soft at the edges but not cooked through.

2. Remove the lid and increase the heat to medium-high. Sprinkle the vegetables with the smoked paprika and stir to mix. Cook, stirring, for 1 minute. Add the water and bring to a boil. Cover and reduce the heat to a simmer. Cook until the potatoes are falling apart and can be easily smashed against the sides of the pot, about 15 minutes.

3. Mash the potatoes into the broth—use an immersion blender if you like your soups smoother. Raise the heat and stir in the shredded kale. Cook until it has turned a bright green and is tender. Stir in the parsley and cook 1 minute more. Serve drizzled with a little extra olive oil.

Ann's Tips

· ⌘ ·

If you cannot find bagged kale, buy 1 large bunch lacinato kale: stack the de-stemmed leaves on top of one another and cut across into ¼-inch strips, keeping your fingers behind the blade.

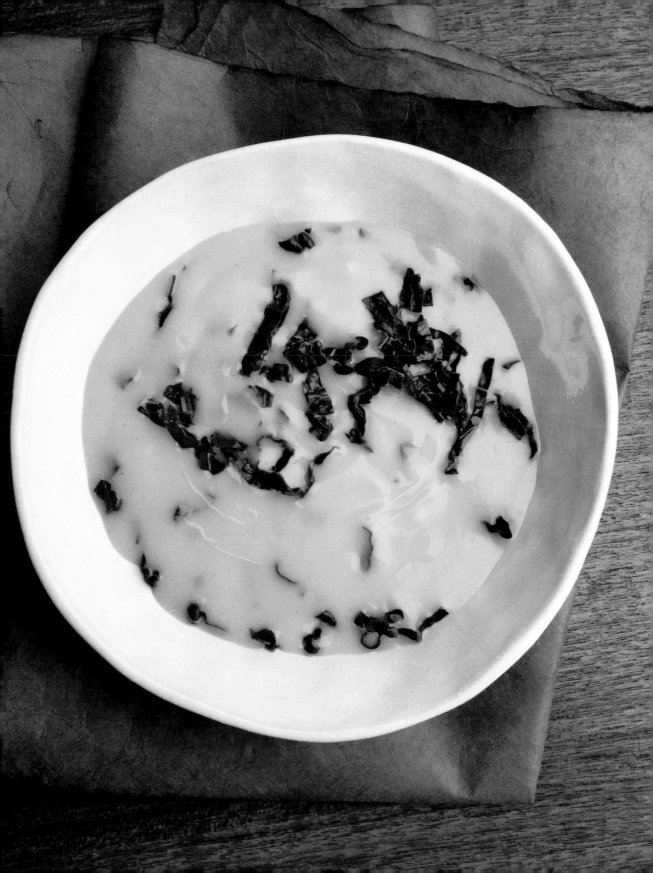

Simple Tuscan Bean Soup with Crunchy Sage Croutons

Meal: Main

Main Ingredients:
Cannellini beans,
Tomatoes

Prep Time: 10 minutes

Cook Time: 45 minutes

SERVES 4 TO 6

HEALTH CONSIDERATIONS: IN TREATMENT; EASY TO SWALLOW; HEALTHY SURVIVORSHIP; NEUTROPENIC DIET

FOOD PREFERENCE: DAIRY-FREE; VEGAN; VEGETARIAN

This is an easy, super-simple pantry soup that you can make right from the cupboard. It gives canned beans the tasty flavor of homemade. If you have Quick Tomato Sauce (page 27) in the freezer, you can even skip step 2. The croutons add a delightful crunch and the beans add some complete protein, but if you don't want to make them, just drizzle the soup with a little of the warm sage-scented oil and scatter crispy sage leaves over the top.

Health Tip

Beans are a great source of protein and fiber and are rich in minerals and B-complex vitamins, particularly folate.

---

4 cups low-sodium vegetable or chicken stock

4 cloves garlic, 2 peeled, smashed, and left whole; 2 thinly sliced lengthwise

6 fresh sage leaves, 2 whole; 4 thinly sliced

2 tablespoons extra-virgin olive oil, divided

1 (28-ounce) can diced tomatoes

Sea salt, to taste

2 (14-ounce) cans of cannellini beans, rinsed and drained

2 (½-inch-thick) slices whole-wheat sourdough bread, crusts trimmed, then cubed (see Ann's Tips, next page)

1. Put the stock, 2 smashed cloves of garlic, 1 teaspoon of olive oil, and the 2 whole sage leaves into a 5-quart Dutch oven or pot. Bring to a boil over high heat and cover. Reduce the heat to medium-low and simmer, covered, for 20 minutes.

2. While the stock is simmering, heat 1 tablespoon of olive oil in a frying pan over medium-high heat. Add half the sliced garlic and cook, stirring until it is golden, about 2 minutes. Add the tomatoes, sprinkle with salt, and cook about 10 minutes, or until they begin to turn orangey-red.

3. Add the beans and tomatoes to the stock. Cook until the beans are soft enough to be smashed against the sides of the pan, 10 to 15 minutes, depending on the brand. The soup should be thick.

4. Meanwhile, make the sage oil: Heat the remaining olive oil in a small sauté pan over medium-high heat. Add the remaining sliced garlic and cook for 1 to 2 minutes, or just until it starts to color. Add the shredded sage and cook until the sage is crisp but not colored, about 2 minutes. Remove the sage from the hot oil, transfer onto a paper towel, and reserve. Discard the garlic.

5. For the croutons: Add the diced bread to the hot sage oil in a single layer, a few cubes at a time—do not crowd the pan. Cook until crisp and brown, and set aside on a paper towel. Repeat with the remaining bread cubes. Sprinkle the croutons and crispy sage on top of the individual bowls as you serve.

If you have made our Basic Beans 2 (page 40), another vegan version would be to omit step 1 and use their broth instead of vegetable stock.

One slice of bread makes enough croutons for 2 or 3 bowls.

Ann's
Tips

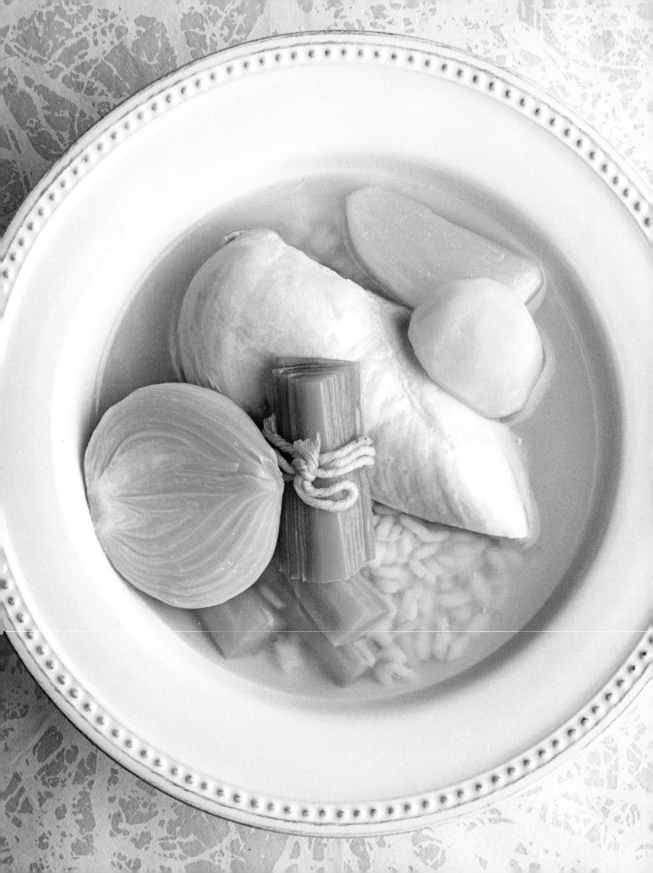

Poached Chicken Pot au Feu (Miracle Chicken)

Meal: Lunch, Dinner

Main Ingredient: Chicken

Prep Time: 20 minutes

Cook Time: 50 minutes

SERVES 4 TO 6

HEALTH CONSIDERATIONS: IN TREATMENT; BLAND DIET; LOW FIBER; GLUTEN-FREE; NEUTROPENIC DIET; HEALTHY SURVIVORSHIP; EASY TO SWALLOW

FOOD PREFERENCE: DAIRY-FREE

My friends call this easy one-pot dish "Miracle Chicken." It's one of my favorite things to eat when I feel tired or run-down. It was a life-saver during chemo. It is basically nourishing, low-fat, invalid food, but it is easy to make and amazingly tasty. The trick is to poach the dish slowly. I use chicken on the bone and always include thighs for extra flavor, but you can use whole, boneless breasts for less mess. If you don't like rice, you can substitute 3 to 4 small, halved, waxy potatoes instead and add them along with the root vegetables in step 3.

2 small yellow onions, peeled and cut in half

8 whole cloves

2 leeks, root ends trimmed off, dark tops reserved

3 medium carrots, peeled

4 pieces organic, free-range skinless chicken on the bone, halved breasts and thighs

4 small white turnips, peeled and quartered

1 bay leaf

½ teaspoon black peppercorns

4 to 6 cups Quick, Rich Chicken Broth (page 24) or water

Sea salt, to taste

1⅓ cups arborio or other short-grain rice

Dijon mustard (optional)

1. Stud each onion half with 2 cloves. Cut the white part of the trimmed leeks into three equal lengths, then in half lengthwise. Set aside. Tie the tender dark tops of the leeks together with a piece of string. Cut the carrots in half, then into quarters lengthwise.

2. Put the chicken into a heavy Dutch oven or other wide pot with a lid. Add just enough water to cover and bring to a boil. As soon as the chicken flesh turns opaque, about 5 minutes, transfer to a plate and discard the water in the pot. Rinse the pot and wipe clean.

3. To the cleaned pot, add the onions, bundled leek greens, carrots, turnips, bay leaf, and peppercorns. Reserve the leek whites. Add enough broth to cover the vegetables completely. Bring to a low simmer, cover, then turn the heat down to medium-low. Gently simmer the vegetables for 10 minutes.

4. Return the chicken to the pot. Tuck it in among the simmering vegetables and top with the reserved leek whites. Sprinkle with a little sea salt and cover. Cook at a simmer over very low heat for about 20 minutes. The chicken should be just cooked and the vegetables tender but not mushy. Taste and adjust seasonings as needed. Add the rice directly to the pot, cover, and cook at a low simmer for 15 minutes or until the rice is al dente. Turn off the heat and let the pot sit, covered, for 10 minutes for the rice to steam and the flavors to develop.

5. To serve, remove the bundled leek greens and discard. Cut the chicken pieces in half. Plate the chicken with half an onion and some carrots, turnips, leek whites, and rice. Spoon stock over the chicken and vegetables. Serve with Dijon mustard on the side, if desired.

Ann's Tips

· ✳ ·

If leeks aren't available, substitute two small celery stalks cut into sticks.

You can cook a whole 3½- to 4-pound chicken this way—ask the butcher to skin it for you. Add the bird back to the pot in step 3 along with the soup vegetables, and increase the simmering time to 20 minutes before adding the leeks in step 4.

Chicken en Papillote with Mustard

Meal: Main

Main Ingredient: Chicken

Prep Time: 20 minutes, plus 30 minutes for marinating

Cook Time: 25 minutes

SERVES 4

HEALTH CONSIDERATIONS: IN TREATMENT; BLAND DIET; LOW FIBER; GLUTEN-FREE; NEUTROPENIC DIET; NAUSEA

FOOD PREFERENCE: DAIRY-FREE

This recipe transforms simple thin-sliced chicken breasts into a total taste treat. The prep can be done while the chicken is marinating, and once the ingredients are assembled and the bag is closed, you will be eating in 25 to 30 minutes, tops. Paper bag cooking is a favorite in our classes. Although at first glance it may seem tricky, people marvel at how easy it is. Anyone can do it. It is an excellent way to get great flavor without too much prep or too much smell, a boon during treatment. It's also perfect for making single portions in one go—think single bag instead of one pot—great if you live alone or there are just two of you to cook for. If you find parchment too tricky to handle, use foil instead.

2 tablespoons Dijon mustard

½ cup plus 2 teaspoons dry white wine such as Pinot Grigio

Sea salt, to taste

¼ teaspoon freshly ground black pepper

4 (3- to 4-ounce) pieces thinly sliced chicken breast (escalopes)

2 tablespoons extra-virgin olive oil

2 large Yukon Gold potatoes, scrubbed and thinly sliced

1 Pink Lady, Braeburn, or other tart-sweet apple, halved, cored, and thinly sliced

2 to 3 sprigs fresh tarragon, leaves stripped

2 medium shallots, thinly sliced

1. Place a rimmed baking sheet in the top third of the oven. Preheat the oven to 425°F. Cut 4 pieces of parchment paper 12 to 18 inches long, or big enough to

comfortably hold the chicken and vegetables when folded. Fold each in half to make a rough square. Set aside (see Ann's Tips, below).

2. In a small bowl, stir together the mustard with the 2 teaspoons of white wine, a pinch of salt, and the pepper. Rub the mixture into the chicken pieces, cover with plastic wrap, and set aside in a cool place to marinate for 30 minutes.

3. After the chicken has marinated, place a parchment square on a work surface. Drizzle 1 teaspoon of olive oil on the bottom half near the crease. Top with a single layer of slightly overlapped potato slices about the same size as the piece of chicken. Sprinkle with a little salt. Add a layer of apple slices, some tarragon leaves, and some shallots. Top with chicken and its marinade. Add another layer of shallots and 3 to 4 slices of potato on top of the chicken. Sprinkle with a little more olive oil, salt, and a grind or two of black pepper.

4. Fold the top of the paper over the chicken and veggies. Starting at the right-hand corner, tightly fold the edges of the paper together to seal the bag. When you get to the left-hand side, leave the corner open. Pour in 2 tablespoons white wine and finish the seal. Set aside. Repeat with the remaining parchment, vegetables, and chicken.

5. Place the bags on the hot baking sheet and bake for 20 minutes. Remove from the oven and let the bags rest for 5 to 10 minutes before opening. Serve with all the juices from the bags.

Ann's Tips

· ✿ ·

Parchment paper comes unbleached or bleached, and in various sizes of precut and cut-as-you-go rolls. I tend to prefer unbleached and cut-as-you-go, usually about 15 inches wide. If you don't bake that often, you can cut the roll to fit the dishes you have, or as here, for the food you are cooking.

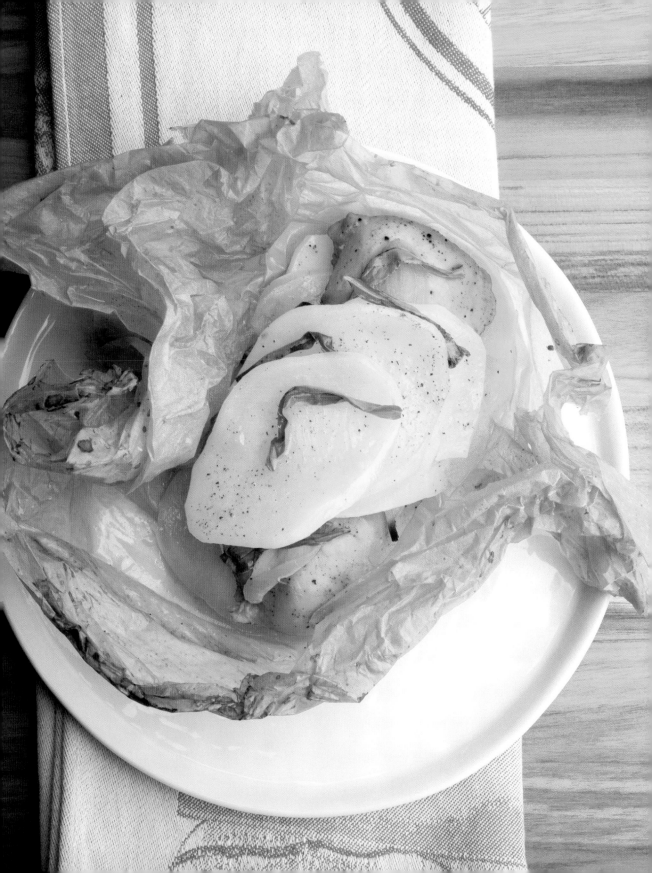

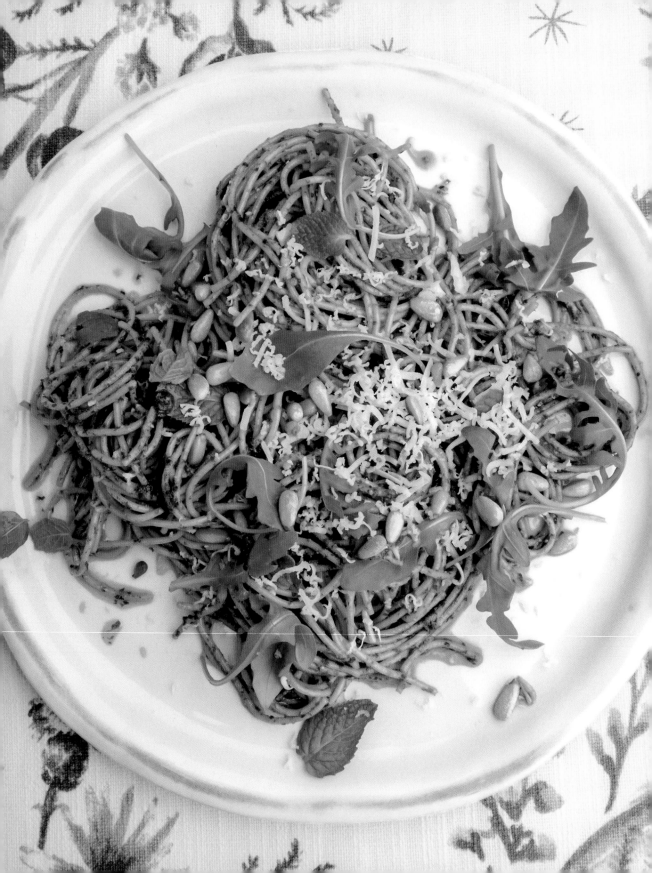

Arugula Pesto with Whole-Wheat Spaghettini

Meal: Basics, Sauces

Main Ingredient: Arugula

Prep Time: 15 minutes

Cook Time: 6 minutes

SERVES 4

HEALTH CONSIDERATIONS: IN TREATMENT; FATIGUE; HEALTHY SURVIVORSHIP

FOOD PREFERENCE: VEGETARIAN

This pesto is a spicy version of the classic Italian raw herb sauce. It gets its spiciness from tangy arugula, and it's best to use the tiny-leaved spicy Italian variety if you can get it, but baby arugula is a perfectly good substitute if you can't. Creamy Pecorino Romano melts to perfection when it hits hot pasta, but it is salty, so don't add any extra salt until the cheese is pulsed into your sauce and you've tasted it. Toss the sauce with quick-cooking whole-wheat spaghettini for a delicious meal in a hurry.

8 ounces whole-wheat spaghettini

Arugula Pesto

MAKES 1½ TO 2 CUPS

2 cloves garlic, peeled and sliced

⅔ cup extra-virgin olive oil, divided

⅓ cup pine nuts

2½ cups washed Italian or baby arugula, loosely packed (see Ann's Tips, next page)

1 cup washed flat-leaf parsley, leaves only, loosely packed

½ cup washed mint leaves, loosely packed

½ cup freshly grated Pecorino Romano cheese

½ cup freshly grated Parmesan cheese

½ teaspoon sea salt, or to taste

Freshly ground black pepper, to taste

1. Set a large pot of water to boil.
2. In a food processor, process the garlic with ⅓ cup of the olive oil. Add the pine nuts and then the arugula and the herbs a handful at a time. Process until finely chopped together.

3. Leaving the motor running, gradually add the remaining olive oil using the feed tube until well blended with the herbs. Add the cheeses and pulse to mix. Taste for salt. Pulse again to mix. Transfer ½ cup pesto into a large bowl and set aside. Reserve the rest for another use or to freeze.

4. Cook the spaghettini in the boiling water for about 30 seconds less than suggested on the package instructions. Drain, reserving ½ cup of the cooking water. Tip the hot pasta on top of the pesto in the bowl. Toss to mix, adding some of the reserved water as you go, 1 tablespoon at a time. This will loosen the pesto and make it more "saucy." The pasta should be just covered in sauce but not swimming in it. Serve immediately with freshly grated Parmesan cheese and a grind or two of black pepper.

Ann's Tips

· ❀ ·

This pesto freezes well. You can use it in many ways: as a relish for fish, chicken, or vegetables; to flavor soups; or as here, a sauce for pasta.

As a rule of thumb, 2 ounces dry weight of pasta is the correct portion size.

Pasta Pomodoro Basilico

HEALTH CONSIDERATIONS: IN TREATMENT; FATIGUE; HIGH FIBER; HIGH CALORIE; GLUTEN-FREE; NEUTROPENIC DIET; HEALTHY SURVIVORSHIP

FOOD PREFERENCE: VEGETARIAN

Meal: Main

Main Ingredients: Whole-wheat pasta, Tomatoes

Prep Time: 10 minutes

Cook Time: 12 to 15 minutes

SERVES 2 TO 3

Who would have thought that something so deeply delicious as this classic dish would be one of the easiest, quickest things to make? Just a few leaves of fresh basil and the simple tomato sauce that I use for nearly every pasta bring to life the taste of an Italian summer. Significantly, its bright acidity is the perfect wake-up for a jaded chemo palate. The trick to this simple sauce is to add the fresh basil right at the end and cook it for just a minute so it can give its full fragrance to the sauce. It's so quick and easy that if you put on a pot of water to boil for the pasta and start the sauce, the sauce will be done before the pasta has finished cooking. *Che bello!*

4 to 6 ounces whole-wheat or gluten-free rigatoni (see Ann's Tips, next page)

2 tablespoons extra-virgin olive oil

1 to 2 cloves garlic, peeled, smashed, and thinly sliced

1 small dried red pepper, seeds removed (optional)

1 (14-ounce) can organic chopped tomatoes (see Ann's Tips, next page)

Sea salt, to taste

1 tablespoon freshly grated Parmesan cheese, plus additional for serving

8 to 10 basil leaves, roughly torn into pieces

1. Bring a large pot of water to a boil over high heat. Cook the pasta for 1 minute less than suggested on the package instructions, then drain and set aside, reserving 1 cup of the cooking water.
2. While the water is heating, heat the oil in a wok or heavy frying pan over medium-high heat. When the oil starts to shimmer a little, add the garlic and

stir-fry until it is just golden, about 2 minutes. Do not let it burn or it will become bitter. If you like a spicy sauce, add the pepper at this time.

3. Add the tomatoes and cook, stirring. (The tomatoes will spit and hiss when they hit the hot oil.) Sprinkle with a little salt. Reduce the heat to medium-low and cook the tomatoes down until they are saucy and an orangey-red color and have reduced by about half, 5 to 8 minutes. Stir the Parmesan cheese into the sauce. If the sauce looks like it's drying out too much, add a little of the reserved pasta water. Taste for salt and adjust as needed.

4. Add the torn basil leaves to the sauce. Stir to wilt, then add the cooked pasta and a little of the reserved pasta water, if needed. Cook, stirring, for 1 minute to coat the pasta with the sauce. Serve immediately with additional freshly grated Parmesan cheese.

Ann's Tips

Allow 2 ounces of dry-weight pasta per person for the perfect portion.

In the summer, when tomatoes are at their peak, use 4 or 5 ripe plum tomatoes, or 1 large ripe beefsteak tomato (about 12 ounces), washed and coarsely chopped, in place of the canned tomatoes.

In the winter, if you can't find fresh basil, use 1 or 2 teaspoons of frozen Arugula Pesto (page 65) or commercial jarred traditional basil pesto.

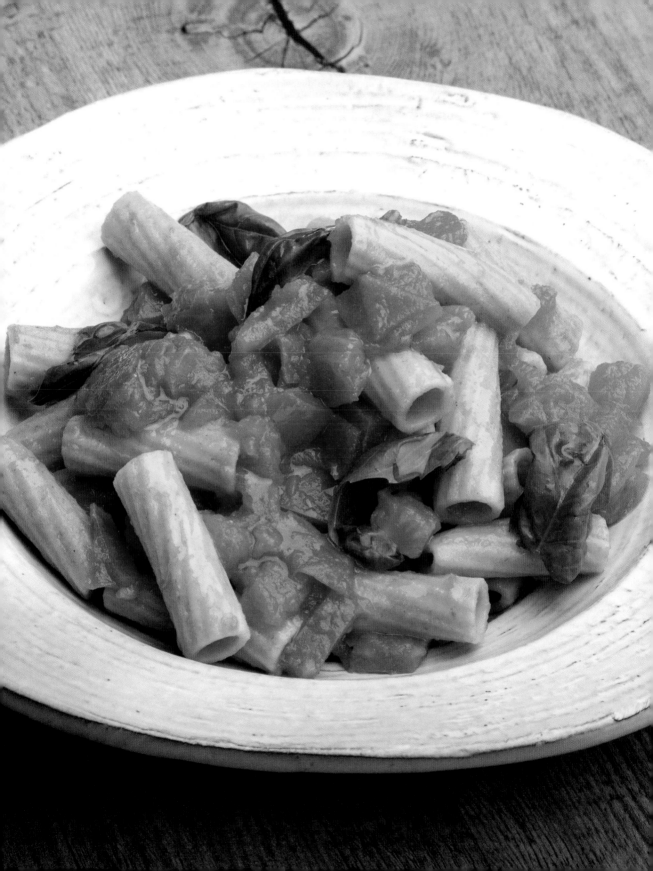

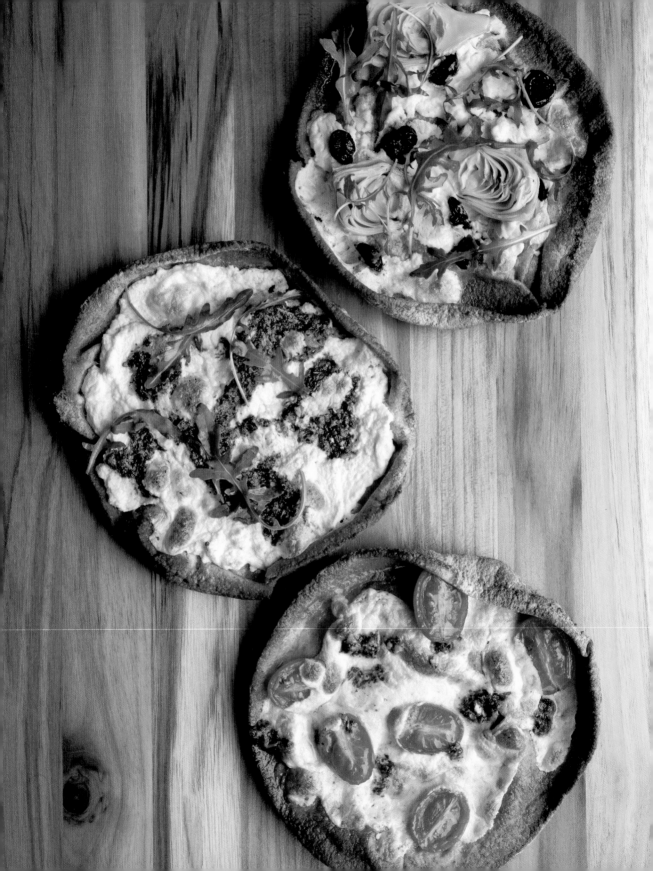

Pita Pizza

HEALTH CONSIDERATIONS: IN TREATMENT; FATIGUE; NEUTROPENIC DIET

FOOD PREFERENCE: VEGETARIAN

These "pizzas" are super quick and simple enough to make in a toaster oven. You can put almost anything on a pizza, and there are more variations for these treats than I can possibly write down here. But these three topping ideas will give you an idea of the variety, and of just how easy and delicious it is to get started.

1 whole-wheat pita bread

½ teaspoon extra-virgin olive oil

For all, preheat the oven or toaster oven to 425°F. Or set the broiler to high and lower the rack.

Tomato and Mozzarella with Basil (a Classic)

2 tablespoons shredded mozzarella or chopped mozzarella bocconcini, divided

2 to 3 cherry tomatoes, rinsed and sliced

1 teaspoon grated Parmesan cheese

2 basil leaves, torn into pieces, or ½ teaspoon pesto

1. Place the pita bread on a baking sheet. Drizzle with the olive oil. Sprinkle with 1 tablespoon of the mozzarella. Scatter the tomato slices on top. Top with the remaining 1 tablespoon mozzarella and the Parmesan. Bake or broil until the cheese has melted and the pita is browned, 5 to 7 minutes. Scatter with basil or drizzle with pesto and eat.

Meal: Mains, Snacks

Main Ingredient: Mozzarella

Prep Time: 10 minutes

Cook Time: 5 to 7 minutes

SERVES 1

Arugula Pesto and Ricotta (Creamy and Light)

1 tablespoon ricotta cheese

1 tablespoon Arugula Pesto (page 65)

1 tablespoon shredded mozzarella or chopped mozzarella bocconcini

1. Place the pita bread on a baking sheet. Drizzle with the olive oil. Spread with the ricotta cheese and scatter with the pesto. Top with the mozzarella. Bake or broil until the cheese has melted and the pita is browned, 5 to 7 minutes. Eat.

Artichoke, Black Olive, and Goat Cheese with Arugula (Salty and Sharp)

1 tablespoon crumbled creamy goat cheese

4 artichoke hearts, frozen or canned, sliced

2 pitted oil-cured black olives, sliced

1 tablespoon shredded mozzarella or chopped mozzarella bocconcini

Arugula leaves

1. Place the pita bread on a baking sheet. Drizzle with the olive oil. Spread with the crumbled goat cheese. Scatter artichokes and olives on top, and sprinkle with the mozzarella. Bake or broil until the cheese has melted and the pita is browned, 5 to 7 minutes. Pile the arugula leaves on top and eat.

Ann's Tips

Pita bread stores brilliantly in the freezer, so just take out and use what you need. If they're not flat enough to use straight from the freezer, thaw them on the stove top for a few minutes to soften before using.

Although I've recommended whole-wheat pita bread, if you are on a bland diet, use regular white-flour pita instead and tailor the toppings to suit your needs, like the ricotta and pesto. No diet should stop us from eating pizza!

Middle Eastern Turkey Burgers

HEALTH CONSIDERATIONS: IN TREATMENT; FATIGUE; LOW FIBER; GLUTEN-FREE; NEUTROPENIC DIET; HEALTHY SURVIVORSHIP

FOOD PREFERENCE: NONE

Eastern Mediterranean cooking has a rich repertoire of spiced meatballs and meat fillings used for savory pastries. These burgers take their cue from this ancient tradition, only instead of lamb, I've used less-fatty ground turkey. Chopped spinach, herbs, and ground spices are the key to these delicious, moist burgers. Although you can make them with fresh spinach, frozen does the job just as well and with a lot less work. This is the kind of convenience food I'm happy to see in the kitchen.

Meal: Main

Main Ingredient: Ground turkey

Prep Time: 20 minutes

Cook Time: 15 to 20 minutes

MAKES 4 TO 6 PATTIES

1 (10-ounce) box frozen leaf spinach (see Ann's Tips, next page)

½ cup chopped cilantro

1 small shallot, minced

1 clove garlic, minced

1 pound ground turkey (see Ann's Tips, next page)

2 tablespoons Greek yogurt

½ teaspoon ground cumin

½ teaspoon ground coriander

½ teaspoon sea salt, or to taste

¼ teaspoon freshly ground black pepper

3 tablespoons extra-virgin olive oil

4 to 6 whole-wheat or gluten-free burger buns, toasted

Spiced Yogurt Sauce (page 231)

4 to 6 pieces lettuce

1 avocado, mashed (optional)

1. Thaw the spinach, squeeze out all excess water using a paper towel, and chop.
2. In a medium bowl, combine the spinach, cilantro, shallot, garlic, turkey, yogurt, cumin, and coriander. Season with salt and pepper. Combine until well blended. Form into 4 patties.

3. Heat the oil in a large skillet over medium heat. Cook the patties until golden brown or until cooked through, 5 to 8 minutes per side. Cover the pan with a lid for the middle 2 to 3 minutes of cooking each side to help cook the burgers through.

4. Serve on burger buns with lettuce, Spiced Yogurt Sauce, and mashed avocado, if desired.

Ann's Tips

· 🗶 ·

Don't use frozen chopped spinach, as it will make the burgers too wet. (Once thawed, it is too hard to get rid of its excess water.) You can, however, use fresh spinach instead of frozen. You will need 4 cups of baby spinach, chopped fine. You can use a food processor to chop the spinach if you have one, but take care not to overchop it—you don't want a puree. Pulse 2 or 3 times only and throw in the rest of the burger ingredients to mix.

These burgers can also be grilled on a stove top or electric grill. Or you can broil them on a low setting or rung.

Prepackaged ground turkey runs from 16 ounces (1 pound) to 20 ounces (1¼ pounds). The amounts of spinach and spice in this recipe will work just fine for both, but you may need to increase the salt to ¾ teaspoon for a 20-ounce pack of meat.

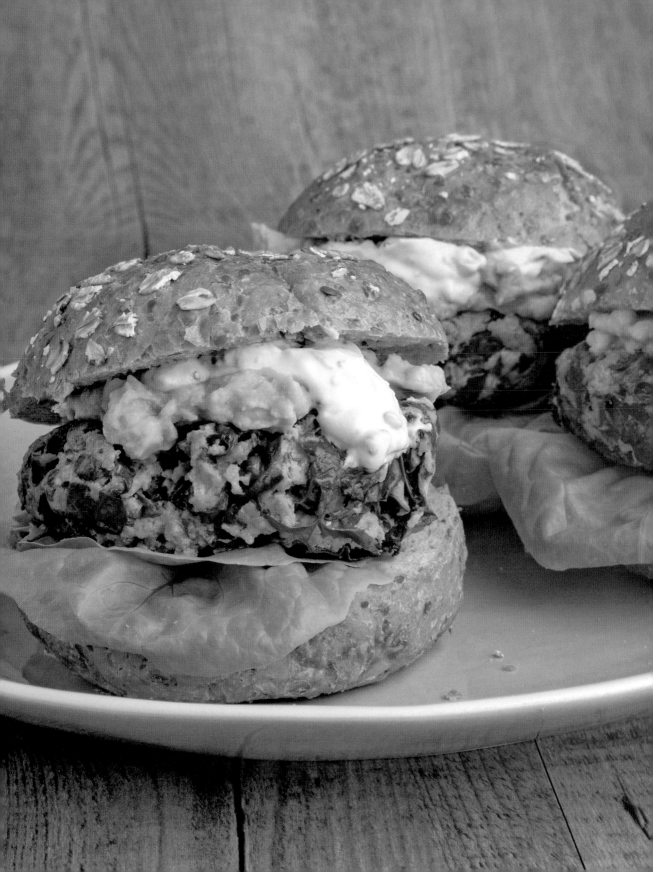

Simple Baked Salmon

Meal: Main

Main Ingredient: Salmon

Prep Time: 10 minutes, plus 30 minutes for marinating

Cook Time: 10 to 12 minutes

SERVES 2

HEALTH CONSIDERATIONS: IN TREATMENT; FATIGUE; BLAND DIET; LOW FIBER; GLUTEN-FREE; NEUTROPENIC DIET; EASY TO SWALLOW

FOOD PREFERENCE: DAIRY-FREE

This salmon couldn't be easier to prepare, and it is really delicious. For something as simple as this, buy the best-quality salmon you can afford—wild-caught Alaskan salmon, if your pocketbook allows. You can use the same marinade to bake the fish, or broil or grill it. I prefer baking because the fish cooks with less odor—a very desirable thing when either you or a family member are going through treatment. Oily fish like salmon can generate too much odor while cooking under the broiler or on the grill, and that can be quite nauseating. In fact, it might be good to save this dish for the up cycle of a chemo regimen, when things are returning to normal.

Juice of ½ lemon

1 teaspoon extra-virgin olive oil

2 to 3 bay leaves, crumbled

1 piece thick salmon fillet, about 10 ounces (see Ann's Tips, next page)

Sea salt, to taste

1. In a dish just big enough to hold the salmon, mix the lemon juice and olive oil together. Add the crumbled bay leaves.
2. Rub the flesh side of the salmon with a little salt and turn it in the marinade until coated, then turn skin-side up and rub a little salt into the skin. Cover with plastic wrap, place in the refrigerator, and allow the salmon to marinate for 30 minutes.
3. While the fish is marinating, preheat the oven to 425°F. Line a baking sheet with parchment paper and place in the upper third of the oven.
4. Remove the salmon from the marinade and place it skin-side down on the hot baking sheet. Quickly spoon any marinade from the dish over the top. Bake for

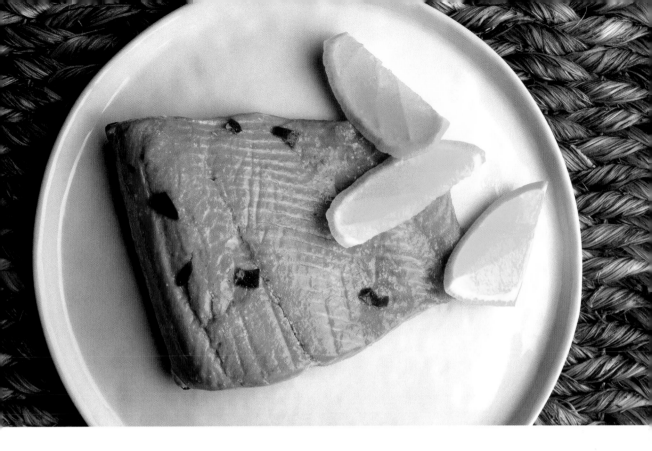

10 to 12 minutes, or until firm when pressed with a fork. The softer the fish, the less cooked it is. Serve immediately.

Ann's Tips

Make sure to get a slice from the thickest part of the fillet. If you don't see it, ask the fishmonger to cut one for you. The pointy tail end is too uneven in thickness to cook evenly.

The rule of thumb is to cook fish 10 minutes per 1 inch of thickness. If you cook a smaller single serving, it will need less baking time, 8 to 10 minutes.

Parchment is key when cooking fish. It makes for easy cleanup with no smelly burnt bits to scrape off your cookware.

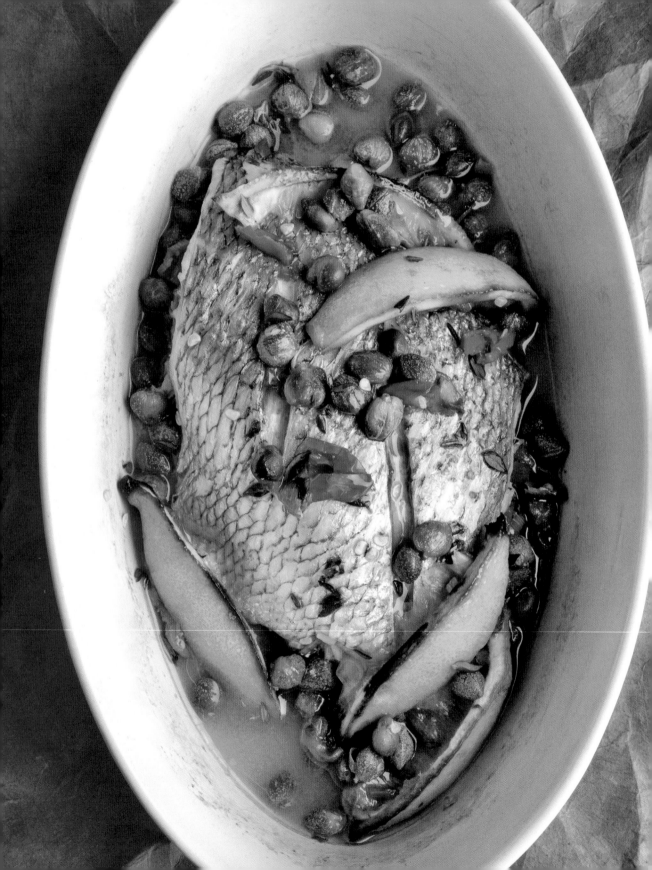

Slow-Baked Fish with Lemon and Capers

Meal: Main

Main Ingredient: Firm white-flesh fish fillets

Prep Time: 10 minutes

Cook Time: 45 minutes

SERVES 4

HEALTH CONSIDERATIONS: IN TREATMENT; FATIGUE; LOW FIBER; GLUTEN-FREE; NEUTROPENIC DIET

FOOD PREFERENCES: DAIRY-FREE

Fish is often cooked quickly in a very hot oven. But not this one; rather, it is slow-cooked in a moderate oven until the flesh just flakes. You will need fillets from a firm, large fish like grouper, halibut, or Chilean sea bass, and since these are expensive fish, it's good to know this method is pretty much foolproof. The flavor of the fish is mild, and the sauce for it is tart and citrusy. For all chili peppers, the heat resides in the seeds and the white pith of the inside ribs, so make sure you remove both for a milder bite. If you're not in the mood for spicy, either put in 1 whole unbroken chili or just leave the chili out altogether. It will still be good.

2 to 3 tablespoons extra-virgin olive oil, divided

1 (2-pound) piece thick, firm whitefish fillet, such as grouper, halibut, or Chilean sea bass, skin on (see Ann's Tips, next page, if you prefer to cook a whole fish)

Sea salt and freshly ground black pepper, to taste

2 to 3 sprigs fresh thyme

3 (½-inch) strips lemon zest

¾ cup dry white wine

Juice of ½ lemon

2 tablespoons capers, drained and rinsed

1 fresh red cayenne chili, seeded and chopped (optional) (see Ann's Tips, next page)

1. Preheat the oven to 350°F. Brush a rectangular 1½-quart (10 x 8 x 1¾ inches) ovenproof dish with olive oil and place on the back of the stove to warm a little as the oven heats up.

2. Using a sharp knife, make 3 slashes across the skin of the fillet. Season both sides with salt and pepper. Place in the prepared baking dish skin-side up and tuck the thyme and lemon zest underneath. Brush the top with the remaining olive oil. Pour in the wine and lemon juice. Bake for 15 minutes.

3. Add the capers and chili, if using, to the pan. Continue to cook for another 25 to 30 minutes, basting occasionally, or until the fish is easily pierced with a fork. Transfer to a warm dish. Spoon the sauce over the fish and serve.

Ann's Tips

· ⚓ ·

To cook a whole fish, choose a couple of 1½-pound snappers, striped bass, or branzinos. Get your fishmonger to clean, scale, and trim the fins from the fish. In step 2, season the fish with salt and pepper inside and out, tuck all the thyme and lemon zest inside the fish's body cavity and brush the top with oil. Add the wine and lemon juice and continue to cook as directed.

Unless you like very spicy foods, shake the seeds out of dried chilies before using and cut the seeds and white pith out of fresh chilies.

Creamy Kale and Apple Salad

HEALTH CONSIDERATIONS: IN TREATMENT; FATIGUE; HIGH FIBER; GLUTEN-FREE; HEALTHY SURVIVORSHIP

FOOD PREFERENCE: VEGETARIAN; NUTS

Kale is one of the superstars of the cancer-fighting cruciferous family. The combination of a tart, creamy dressing and sweet apples in this simple, Waldorf-style salad showcases raw kale to its best advantage, and it tastes nicely decadent to boot. Because kale is not as delicate as softer salad greens like lettuce, it actually improves from sitting in the dressing. Make this salad ahead of time and let it sit in the fridge until you're ready to eat.

Meal: Main

Main Ingredient: Kale

Prep Time: 25 minutes

Cook Time: 0 minutes

SERVES 4

Health Tip

This dressing contains probiotic yogurt, so if you are on a neutropenic diet, check with your doctor or registered dietician that it's safe for you to eat.

Creamy Mustard Vinaigrette
MAKES ABOUT ½ CUP

1 tablespoon cider vinegar

1 tablespoon Dijon mustard

Sea salt and freshly ground black pepper, to taste

3 tablespoons extra-virgin olive oil

2 tablespoons plain whole milk or 2% Greek yogurt

1 tablespoon water, as needed

Salad

1 Golden Delicious apple, quartered, cored, and thinly sliced (see Ann's Tips, next page)

2 scallions, white and pale green parts only

1 bunch lacinato kale, stems stripped and leaves thinly sliced (see Ann's Tips, next page)

¼ cup walnuts, toasted and coarsely chopped, for garnish

1. Make the dressing: In a large salad bowl, whisk together the cider vinegar, mustard, salt, and pepper. Whisk in the olive oil, then the Greek yogurt. Taste for sharpness and seasoning. Add water, 1 teaspoon at a time, if the dressing is too sharp for your palate. If not using straightaway, store the dressing in a container in the fridge, where it will keep for up to 3 days.
2. Toss the apples and scallions into the dressing and pile the kale on top with half the walnuts. Toss together until the kale is well coated in dressing. Scatter with the remaining walnuts. Cover and refrigerate until ready to serve.

Ann's Tips

· ✦ ·

To shred kale, stack about one-third of the stripped leaves on top of one another and tightly roll up. Thinly slice through the roll. The result is a pile of shredded kale. Repeat with the remaining leaves. In culinary terms, this shredding is called a chiffonade.

To stop sliced apples from going brown, squeeze ¼ lemon into a medium bowl of cold water and swish it around. Place apple slices directly into the water.

I always choose to use whole-milk Greek yogurt and eat less of it, but if you want to cut down further on the fat, use 2% rather than fat-free, as it's more natural. Fat-free yogurt has extra carbs added to give it a better mouthfeel.

The highest-quality yogurts are made from milk and bacteria called probiotics, which assist in maintaining a healthy gut and overall well-being. Check the ingredients when purchasing yogurt.

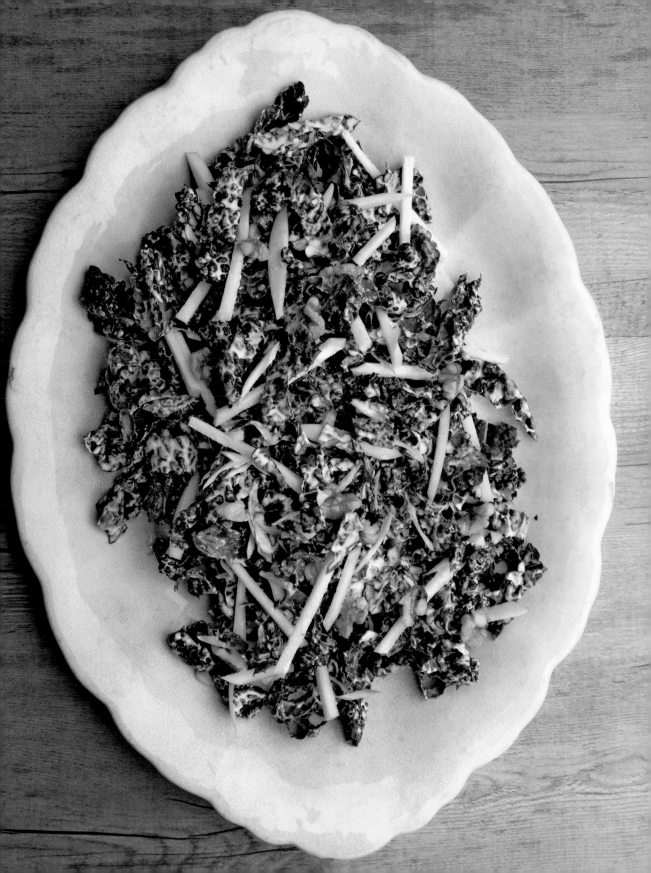

Easy Potato Salad

Meal: Side

Main Ingredient: Potatoes

Prep Time: 20 minutes

Cook Time: 20 minutes

SERVES 4 TO 6

HEALTH CONSIDERATIONS: IN TREATMENT; FATIGUE; GLUTEN-FREE; HEALTHY SURVIVORSHIP

FOOD PREFERENCE: VEGETARIAN

I'm not a great fan of potatoes in heavy mayonnaise dressings. I much prefer them tossed in lighter vinaigrettes. This potato salad is made with Creamy Mustard Vinaigrette and is the best of both worlds. The vinaigrette-based dressing is light but creamy and makes an excellent substitute for mayonnaise. Tossed with chives and tarragon, which add gorgeous fresh flavor, this is one delicious salad. And with two different-color potatoes, it's good to look at, too.

Health Tip

This dressing contains probiotic yogurt, so if you are on a neutropenic diet, check with your doctor or a registered dietician that it's safe for you to eat.

½ pound small Yukon Gold potatoes, washed and quartered

½ pound small Red Bliss potatoes, washed and quartered

1 stalk celery, finely diced

¼ cup sliced chives (about ½ bunch)

½ cup Creamy Mustard Vinaigrette (page 81)

2 sprigs tarragon, leaves stripped and roughly chopped

1. Put the potatoes into a small saucepan. Add water to just cover. Bring to a boil and cook until the potatoes are soft but still hold their shape, 15 to 20 minutes. Drain and set aside. This can be done up to a day ahead of time, just keep the potatoes refrigerated and bring them to room temperature before assembling the salad.

2. Meanwhile, in a salad bowl, mix together the celery, chives, and Creamy Mustard Vinaigrette.

3. Transfer the potatoes to the bowl and toss with the dressing. Cover and set aside in a cool place for 30 minutes to allow the flavors to blend. Just before serving, sprinkle with the chopped tarragon.

If you toss the potatoes in the dressing while still warm, they will quickly absorb the dressing and all its flavors.

If your doc won't let you eat yogurt, use Mustard Vinaigrette (page 291).

Ann's Tips

· ☖ ·

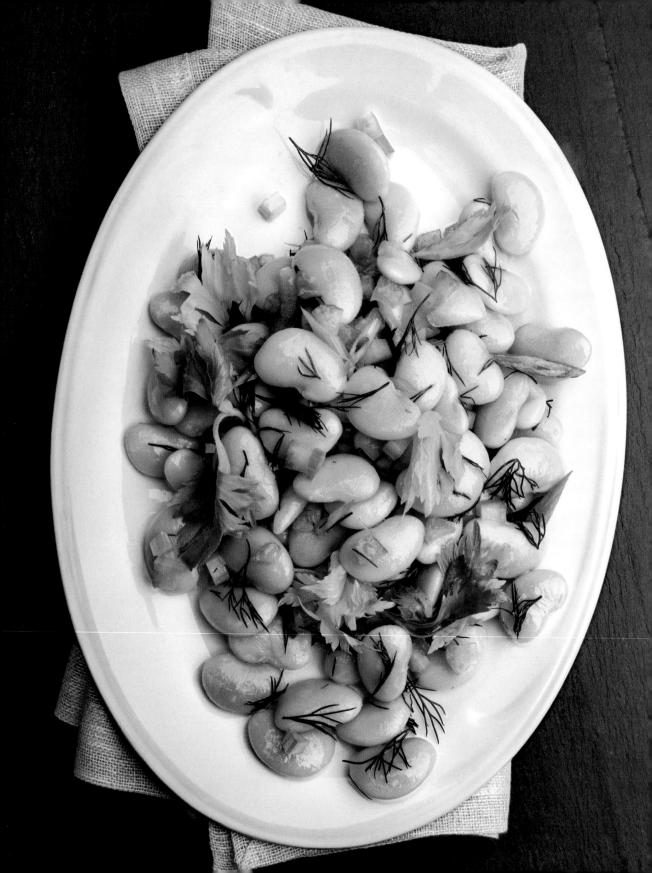

Herby Broad Bean Salad

HEALTH CONSIDERATIONS: GLUTEN-FREE; IN TREATMENT; HIGH FIBER; HEALTHY SURVIVORSHIP; NAUSEA; FATIGUE

FOOD PREFERENCE: DAIRY-FREE; VEGAN; VEGETARIAN

Meal: Salads, Sides

Main Ingredient: Broad beans

Prep Time: 15 minutes, plus 30 minutes resting time

Cook Time: 0 minutes

SERVES 6 TO 8

Whether you call them *habas grandes*, gigantes, or broad beans, these large white lima beans are popular in Greek, Turkish, and Spanish cuisines. They are easy to find in the international aisle of most supermarkets, usually in the Goya section. Their creamy flavor is wonderful with salty celery, especially if it still has its rich dark green leaves. Added to the salad, the leaves can add a lot of flavor. If they're missing, flat-leaf parsley is a good substitute.

3 tablespoons extra-virgin olive oil, plus extra for drizzling

1 tablespoon lemon juice

½ teaspoon sea salt, or to taste

2 stalks celery, finely diced, leaves reserved if they are dark green and vibrant (see Ann's Tips, next page)

2 scallions, white parts only, minced

2 tablespoons chopped fresh dill

2 (14-ounce) cans broad beans (*habas grandes*), drained and rinsed

1. In a medium bowl, beat the oil and lemon juice together with the salt. Stir in the celery, scallions, and dill and mix well.
2. Tear the celery leaves into pieces. Gently stir the celery leaves and beans into the salad until the beans are coated with dressing. Drizzle a little extra oil over the salad if the beans seem dry. Set aside for 30 minutes to allow the flavors to blend. Serve the salad at room temperature.

Ann's
Tips

⚶

Because of pesticide use, celery is one of the "Dirty Dozen" vegetables that should always be bought organic if possible. For more information on the "Dirty Dozen" list, go to the Environmental Working Group's website, ewg.org.

If you can't find broad beans, use cannellini. Navy beans are too small for this recipe.

Simple Roasted Savoy Cabbage

HEALTH CONSIDERATIONS: IN TREATMENT; FATIGUE; BLAND DIET; GLUTEN-FREE; NEUTROPENIC DIET; HEALTHY SURVIVORSHIP

FOOD PREFERENCE: DAIRY-FREE; VEGAN; VEGETARIAN

Meal: Side

Main Ingredient: Cabbage

Prep Time: 10 minutes

Cook Time: 15 minutes

SERVES 4 TO 6

Cabbage is bursting with cancer-protecting phytonutrients. Sadly, cabbage is often so badly treated in the kitchen that many of us never choose to eat it. No more! This fast, easy way to cook cabbage is a game changer. Roasting brings out the sweetness of this hearty vegetable in a way that is both simple and delicious. It will turn haters into lovers.

1 small head savoy cabbage, stem and any damaged tough outer leaves removed

2 tablespoons plus 2 teaspoons extra-virgin olive oil, divided

Sea salt, to taste

4 (15-inch) squares parchment or foil

1. Preheat the oven to 400°F. Place a baking sheet on a rack set in the upper third of the oven.
2. Quarter the cabbage and remove the hard core. Cut each quarter into thick slices, about 1 inch wide.
3. Lay one sheet of parchment or foil on your work surface. Drizzle the upper half with 1 teaspoon of the olive oil and cover with one sliced cabbage quarter, spreading the slices a little. Drizzle another teaspoon of oil over them and sprinkle with salt. Fold the bottom side of the parchment over the cabbage and seal the edges by folding. Repeat with the remaining ingredients.
4. Remove the hot baking sheet from the oven and set the packets of cabbage onto it. Return immediately to the oven and bake for 10 to 15 minutes, or until the cabbage is soft and slightly colored around the edges. Remove from the oven and let sit to steam for 5 minutes. Serve piping-hot.

The packet dimensions here comfortably hold one-quarter of a small cabbage. Don't be tempted to overload them. The cabbage won't cook as quickly or as evenly. And don't open the packets until the 5-minute steaming time is up. The steaming just finishes the cooking.

If it's easier for you to handle, use foil for the packets. In the summer, my friend Cyd Cort puts her cabbage in foil packets directly onto the grill. The cabbage may get a little charred, but it's so good.

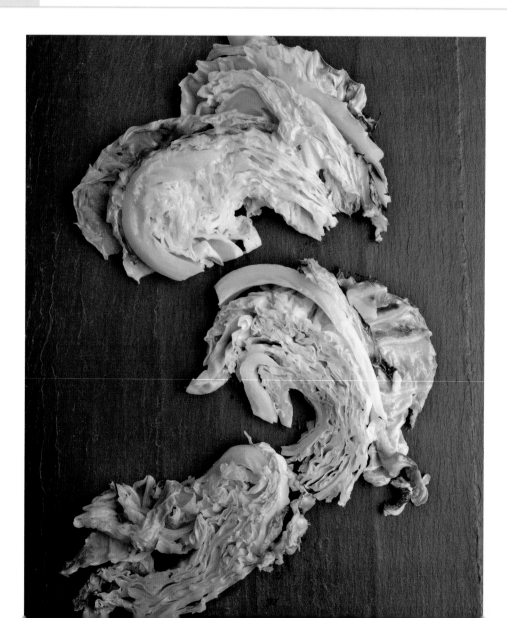

Mint and Cucumber Cooler

HEALTH CONSIDERATIONS: BLAND DIET; GLUTEN-FREE; IN TREATMENT; LOW FIBER; HEALTHY SURVIVORSHIP; NAUSEA; FATIGUE

FOOD PREFERENCE: DAIRY-FREE; VEGAN; VEGETARIAN

Meal: Snacks, Beverages

Main Ingredients: Cucumber, Mint

Prep Time: 5 minutes

Cook Time: 0 minutes

SERVES 6

Because water can taste metallic during treatment, it's tempting to drink a lot of sugary beverages. Infusing water can be a great way to hydrate healthily. Cucumber water is wonderfully refreshing. I added mint to it during my treatment and discovered I'd created an everyday drink that revived my chemo palate and made water drinkable again. If you like the tickle of fizz in your drinks, check out Ann's Tips, below.

1 large cucumber, peeled and sliced

2 sprigs peppermint

1 teaspoon lemon juice

1 quart cool filtered water

Ice cubes, to taste

1. In a large nonreactive jug, combine the cucumber slices, mint, and lemon juice and add enough water to fill the jug. Cover the opening with plastic wrap and let chill in the fridge for 30 minutes to 1 hour, to infuse the water.
2. Serve over ice.

Ann's Tips

To add some fizz, fill a glass halfway with Mint and Cucumber Cooler, add some ice, and top up with plain seltzer.

Microwave Gingered Pears

Meal: Dessert

Main Ingredient: Pears, Ginger

Prep Time: 15 minutes, plus 5 to 10 minutes for steaming

Cook Time: 3 minutes

SERVES 1 OR 2

HEALTH CONSIDERATIONS: BLAND DIET; GLUTEN-FREE; IN TREATMENT; LOW FIBER; EASY TO SWALLOW; NAUSEA; NEUTROPENIC DIET

FOOD PREFERENCE: DAIRY-FREE; VEGAN; VEGETARIAN

This quick and totally delicious recipe is a way to use your microwave for something other than nuking coffee or reheating soup. It's just pears and a little grated ginger. If the pears are very ripe, you may not even need the sugar. This is basically a single or double serving, but if you want to make more, just multiply the ingredients by the number of pears used. However, go easy on the amount of water you add, as the pears will make a lot of steam and a lot of juice.

1 ripe Bosc or Anjou pear, peeled and halved

½ teaspoon grated fresh gingerroot

1 teaspoon fine granulated cane sugar (see Ann's Tips, next page)

1 tablespoon water

1. Carefully scoop out the pear core with a teaspoon, making sure all the seeds are gone. This will leave a little hollow in the pear. Trim out the hard flower end, too.

2. Lay the pears, cut-side up, in a shallow microwave-safe glass or ceramic dish. Sprinkle the cut sides of the pear halves with the ginger, then the sugar. Add the water to the bottom of the dish. Cover with a microwave-safe glass or ceramic plate.

3. Microwave on high for 2 minutes. Carefully remove the dish from the microwave (the plate and dish will be hot, and the pears will have made a lot of juice). Remove the top plate and turn the pears over, spooning the accumulated juices on top. Cover, return to the microwave, and cook for 1 minute more. Once the cooking is done, leave in the oven to steam for 5 to 10 minutes. Remove the dish

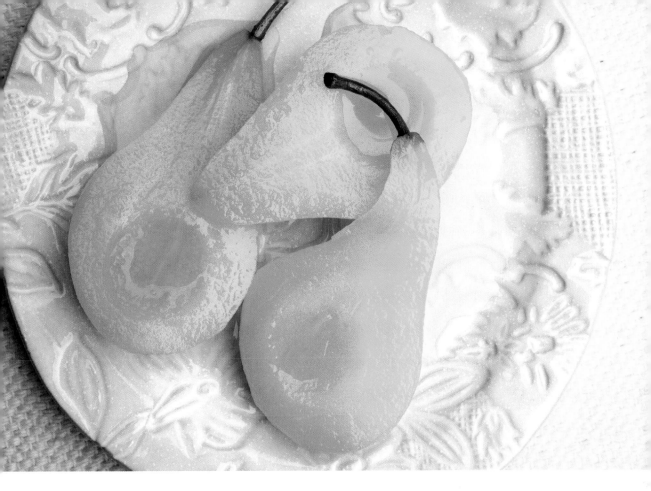

from the microwave and allow the pears to cool. Serve chilled or at room temperature with juices spooned over them.

When cooking in the microwave, always use glass or ceramic containers. I find it useful to set the bowls or plates with the fruit in them on a larger plate or some parchment paper. That way, if the fruit juice boils over, as it sometimes does, cleanup is *much* easier.

If you are preparing several pears at once, drop them into lemon water once they are peeled to keep them from turning brown.

Ann's Tips

· ✲ ·

Soothing

. . . ✛ . . .

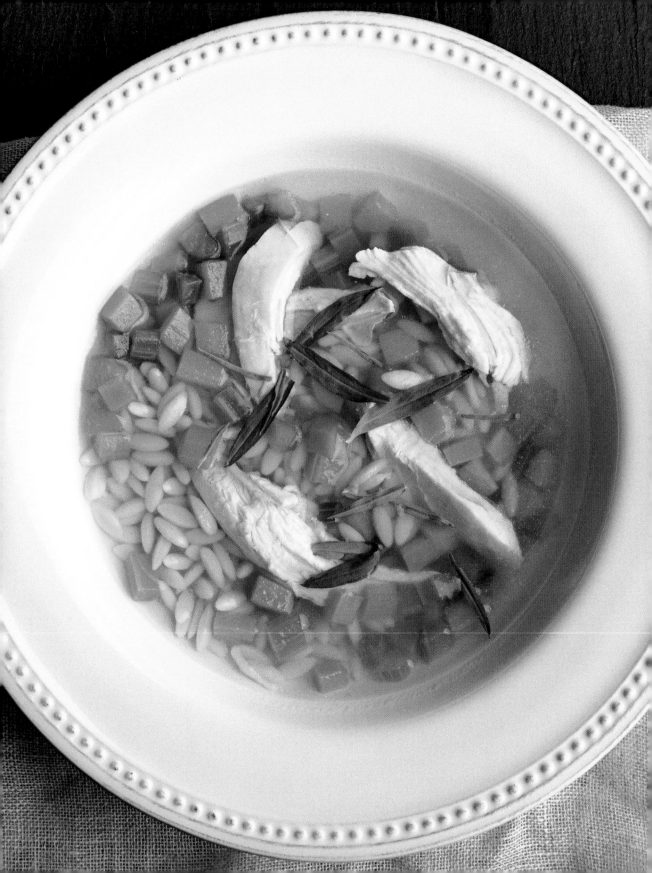

My chemotherapy treatment could make me feel unbelievably awful. There were days when all I could do was lie down like a beached whale and wait for the misery to pass. At times like this, all I wanted to eat was the invalid food that my mum would make me when I was sick as a child, like potato rice soup or poached chicken. These were meals that were comforting and bland, and not too strong smelling as they cooked—in a word, soothing.

Although soothing food can be the simple, homey food I craved, there are also the clinical bland and low-fiber diets that take "bland" woefully well beyond the meaning of the word itself. These diets are designed to ease stress on the digestive tract after a bout of irritable bowel syndrome (IBS), or to help digestion recover after major surgery or during chemo and radiation treatment. But for caretakers and patients alike, the restrictions of these diets can be difficult to cope with. And for patients who have had radiation to the head and neck, only the slippiest of foods can be sipped on.

These soothing foods—white rice, white pastas, potatoes, dairy, no whole grains—can seem contradictory to the accepted norms of good nutrition. And tasteless as well: onions and garlic have to be used sparingly, if at all; vegetables must be steamed or boiled; no spices; nothing that is too acidic or has small seeds. Tomatoes, anyone? Nope. And reduced fat is recommended, too, so no sautéed or fried foods, and all dairy has to be low- or no-fat, except when a sore throat demands fat to help make food easier to swallow. Even members of the mighty cruciferous family such as kale and cabbage have to take a backseat if their fiber isn't well tolerated. But don't worry. Comforting solutions are on the way. It's possible to eat well, and even deliciously, despite the restrictions.

HELPFUL HINTS

As a rule of thumb, it's less stressful on the system to eat frequent small meals rather than the traditional three squares, so portion your food accordingly. And don't hesitate to experiment to see which vegetables your system tolerates best. Introduce them in small amounts to a meal and you'll soon find out. Learn from your body.

COOKING TIPS

It can be helpful to make some small tweaks in your cooking methods, and to your pantry. Here are some basics that may help:

- Use a silicone vegetable steamer to steam veggies. Silicone doesn't hold heat, making it a lot easier to handle than the usual metal rosette steamers.
- To cut down on fat, sauté with stock instead of oil. I think this is easiest to do in a wok.
- If allowed, add onions and garlic, peeled and whole, to stocks or soups to add flavor. Remove them before either blending or serving.
- Try using a pinch of asafetida to replace the flavor of garlic and onions. This pungent spice has been used in India as a garlic and onion substitute for millennia, particularly in aristocratic Brahmin cooking, which doesn't allow the use of either.

Tarragon and Lemon Chicken Soup with Orzo

Meal: Soup

Main Ingredient: Chicken

Prep Time: 20 minutes

Cook Time: 55 minutes

SERVES 6

HEALTH CONSIDERATIONS: IN TREATMENT; NAUSEA; BLAND DIET; HEALTHY SURVIVORSHIP; LOW FIBER; NEUTROPENIC DIET

FOOD PREFERENCE: DAIRY-FREE

Chicken soup is the best when you're feeling low, an all-too-common state during cancer treatment. This version of the classic is as soothing as it is delicious. To get the delicate anise backnotes that make this simple soup so very good, you're going to need to use fresh tarragon; dry just won't do it, since the flavor of soft-leaved herbs like tarragon, parsley, and basil doesn't survive the drying process well. I never cared for tarragon until I tasted it fresh, and now it's a firm favorite.

2 teaspoons extra-virgin olive oil

1 medium onion, chopped

2 stalks celery, cut into ¼-inch dice

2 medium carrots, peeled and cut into ¼-inch dice

Sea salt and freshly ground black pepper, to taste

6 cups water

2 sprigs tarragon

1 (2-inch) piece lemon peel

1¼ pounds skinless, bone-in chicken breasts

½ cup orzo

Juice of ½ lemon

2 teaspoons tarragon leaves, chopped, for garnish

1. In a heavy-bottomed pot with a lid, heat the olive oil over medium heat. Add the onion, celery, carrots, and a sprinkle of salt. Cover and cook, stirring occasionally, for 5 to 8 minutes or until the onion is translucent; do not let it brown.

2. Add the water, tarragon, lemon peel, and chicken. Bring to a boil, then reduce the heat and let simmer for at least 40 minutes, skimming any foam or fat that surfaces. Add a little water if the soup has reduced by more than 1 inch.

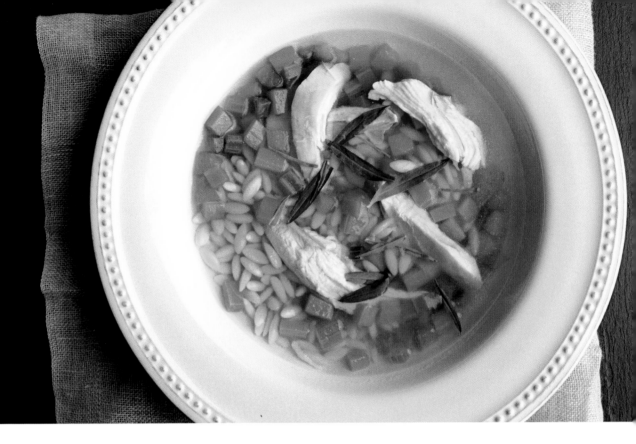

3. Remove the chicken and place into a bowl; allow to cool slightly. Shred the meat and discard the bones. Return the chicken meat to the soup, bring to a boil, then add in the orzo. Boil for 7 minutes, then stir in the lemon juice. Taste for seasonings, then turn off the heat. Ladle into bowls and serve with a sprinkling of fresh tarragon.

Ann's Tips

If you can't find fresh tarragon, julienne the leaves from a sprig of fresh basil or mint. It won't be the same taste, but it will still be a lot better than using dried herbs.

If you are following a neutropenic diet, cook the fresh tarragon in the soup for a couple of minutes before serving.

Stracciatella

HEALTH CONSIDERATIONS: IN TREATMENT; FATIGUE; EASY TO SWALLOW; BLAND DIET; LOW FIBER; NEUTROPENIC DIET; HEALTHY SURVIVORSHIP

FOOD PREFERENCE: NONE

Meal: Lunch, Dinner

Main Ingredients: Chicken or turkey broth, Eggs

Prep Time: 5 minutes

Cook Time: 15 minutes

SERVES 4

Stracciatella is a wonderful word, and a wonderful, nourishing soup for anyone who is feeling tired or low from treatment and wants something easy to digest. The name in Italian literally means "rags," because the stream of beaten egg that gradually gets drizzled in sets into "rags" the instant it hits the simmering broth. My grandma would make it for us when we were sick. Traditionally, the soup is just broth, eggs, and cheese, but she would also add a handful of *stelline* (pasta shaped into tiny little stars) to the broth, which I loved as a child and still do. It's a comment on how easy this soup is to make that when I was a student, I would throw it together whenever I wanted something fast. Of course, I used canned broth or even a stock cube, but this soup is a perfect vehicle for homemade chicken or turkey stock. For extra nutrition and taste, I often throw in a handful of baby arugula. It's quite delicious.

6 cups good low-sodium chicken or turkey broth (Homemade is best! See page 24.)

3 to 4 tablespoons tiny soup pasta, such as orzo, pastina, stelline, or ditalini

2 tablespoons freshly grated Parmesan cheese, divided

2 large eggs (antibiotic-free), beaten well

1 cup loosely packed baby arugula (optional)

Sea salt and freshly ground black pepper, to taste

1. In a large pot, bring the broth to a boil, then reduce the heat until it is at a simmer. Add the pasta and cook for 1 minute less than the time indicated on the package.

2. While the pasta is cooking, beat 1 tablespoon of the Parmesan cheese into the eggs and set aside, then sprinkle the remaining 1 tablespoon of cheese into the broth, stirring until it melts.

3. Two minutes before the pasta has finished cooking, stir the simmering broth to create a swirling circular movement. Using a fork, gradually drizzle in the eggs. They will harden into raggedy strips as soon as they come into contact with the broth. Don't pour the eggs in too fast or you won't get the delicate "rag" effect.

4. Stir in the arugula, if using, and cook until it has just wilted, about 1 minute. Taste for seasonings and serve immediately.

Ann's Tips

· ✦ ·

If you're not using homemade broth, taste-test to find the store brand you like best—it's important for a simple soup like this. Look for a clear broth. The orangey ones tend to have too much carrot. Check out the kosher brands; I find that some of these have the best flavor.

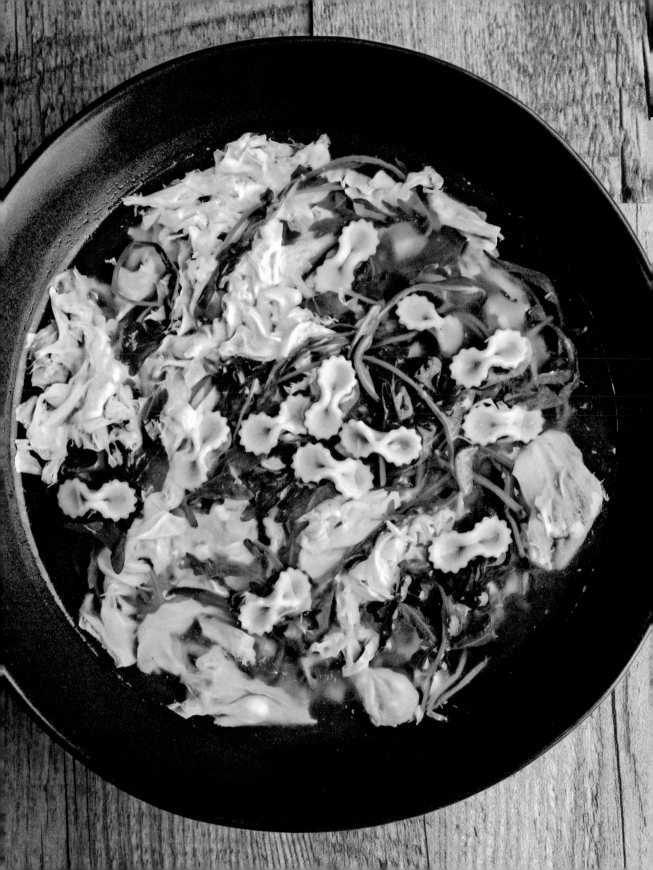

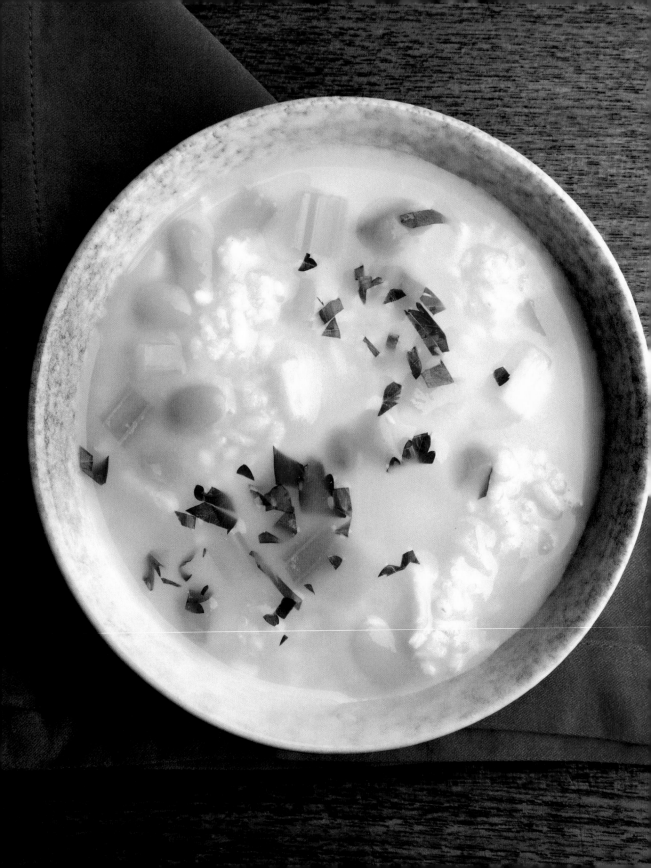

Kohlrabi Rice Soup

HEALTH CONSIDERATIONS: IN TREATMENT; EASY TO SWALLOW; NAUSEA; BLAND DIET; GLUTEN-FREE; NEUTROPENIC DIET; HEALTHY SURVIVORSHIP

FOOD PREFERENCE: VEGETARIAN

Meal: Main

Main Ingredients: Kohlrabi, Arborio rice

Prep Time: 15 to 20 minutes

Cook Time: 40 minutes

SERVES 6 TO 8

This soup is easy to make, easy to cook, and delicious to eat. Kohlrabi is a member of the cancer-bashing cruciferous family, but it is one of those vegetables that can look quite alien until you get to know it. Thanks to the arborio rice, this soup is a great introduction to kohlrabi's sweet flavor. Parmesan cheese is a natural flavor enhancer, so if you don't have a rind handy, stir in 1 tablespoon of grated Parmesan cheese with the lima beans. If you're up for a little kick, drizzle a teaspoon of peppery Arugula Pesto (page 65) over your soup before eating.

1 tablespoon extra-virgin olive oil

3 or 4 medium kohlrabi bulbs, cut into ½-inch dice, leaves reserved, de-stemmed, and shredded (optional)

3 stalks celery, diced (see Ann's Tips, next page)

1 medium onion, diced

Sea salt and freshly ground black pepper, to taste

½ cup arborio rice

4 cloves garlic, minced

6 to 8 cups low-sodium Quick, Rich Chicken Broth (page 24) or Basic Vegetable Broth (page 21)

1 (1-inch) piece Parmesan rind (optional)

1 cup frozen baby lima beans

2 tablespoons roughly chopped parsley (see Ann's Tips, next page)

1. In a heavy pot, heat the olive oil over medium-high heat.
2. Add the kohlrabi, celery, and onion. Sprinkle with salt. Cook, stirring, for 1 minute to coat with oil, then lower the heat and cover. Gently cook the vegetables, stirring occasionally, until the onion is translucent, 8 to 10 minutes. Stir in the rice and garlic and cook, stirring, until you can smell the garlic's aroma, about 2 minutes.

3. Add the broth and bring to a boil. Add the Parmesan rind, if using, and simmer for 30 minutes, or until the vegetables are very tender. Add the lima beans and cook for 2 minutes more, or until they are tender. Taste for seasoning and remove the Parmesan rind. You can either discard it or dice it and return it to the soup. Stir in the parsley and remove the soup from the heat. If you are following a neutropenic diet, cook the parsley in the soup a few minutes longer. Serve immediately.

Ann's Tips

· 🦅 ·

If your celery has a head of dark green leaves, chop and add them to the soup in place of the parsley. Celery leaves add wonderful flavor.

Celery is one of the vegetables best bought organic because of overzealous pesticide use. (For others in this category, check the Environmental Working Group's "Dirty Dozen" list. The good news is that there's a "Clean 15.")

Kohlrabi leaves can be cooked like kale or cabbage. They are quite tender, so strip them from their tough stalks before cooking them. For this soup, the shredded leaves can be added to the soup in step 3, about 5 minutes before the lima beans.

Roasted Carrot Soup
with Tahini

Meal: Main, Soup

Main Ingredients: Carrots, Tahini

Prep Time: 20 minutes

Cook Time: 90 minutes

SERVES 4 TO 6

HEALTH CONSIDERATIONS: IN TREATMENT; FATIGUE; EASY TO SWALLOW; HIGH FIBER; GLUTEN-FREE; NEUTROPENIC DIET; HEALTHY SURVIVORSHIP

FOOD PREFERENCE: DAIRY-FREE; VEGAN; VEGETARIAN; NUTS

This soup is sweetly delicious, creamy, and completely vegan. The cook time may look long, but once you've roasted the carrots, it goes fast. In fact, if you cook the carrots ahead of time and set them aside to use for this, you could have this soothing soup on the table in 40 minutes. It's important to peel the carrots, even though it takes away fiber. This will help them to caramelize and sweeten as they roast.

Health Tip

Although not a tree nut, the sesame seeds that tahini is made from can trigger allergic reactions, so be careful. Sunflower seed butter can be used as a substitute.

2 pounds carrots, rinsed, peeled, and cut into 3-inch pieces

2 tablespoons extra-virgin olive oil, divided

Sea salt and freshly ground black pepper, to taste

1 medium onion, diced

1 bay leaf

1 tablespoon peeled, grated fresh gingerroot, divided

5 to 6 cups Basic Vegetable Broth (page 21) or water

¼ cup tahini

2 tablespoons chopped fresh cilantro

Sweet paprika, for garnish

1. Preheat the oven to 375°F. Line a baking sheet with parchment paper and set aside.
2. Toss the carrots with 1 tablespoon of the olive oil and salt and pepper to taste. Spread onto the prepared baking sheet and roast, turning halfway through, until well browned, tender, and blistered in some areas, about 1 hour.
3. Heat the remaining 1 tablespoon of olive oil in a pot over medium heat. Add the onion, bay leaf, and a sprinkling of salt. Cook until the onion turns translucent, 4 to 5 minutes. Stir in ½ tablespoon of the ginger. Continue to cook for 2 to 3 minutes more, or until the onion begins to brown.
4. Add the roasted carrots and broth. Bring to a boil, then reduce the heat and simmer for at least 30 minutes, or until the carrots are falling apart.
5. Remove the bay leaf. Puree the soup in batches in a blender. (Use caution when blending hot liquids; see page 11). Alternatively, you can use an immersion blender. Return the soup to the pot. Stir in the tahini and the remaining ½ tablespoon of ginger and taste for salt. Bring to a low simmer and cook for 1 minute to heat through. Serve with a dusting of chopped cilantro and paprika.

Ann's Tips

This dish is a great way to repurpose leftovers of other roasted vegetables—think roasted parsnips or beets instead of carrots. Their inherent roasted sweetness would be perfect for this soup. Just go straight to step 3 and get cooking. If you want to use carrots or if you are roasting root vegetables to go with, say, quinoa, as a side, add some extra carrots and set them aside to make this dish.

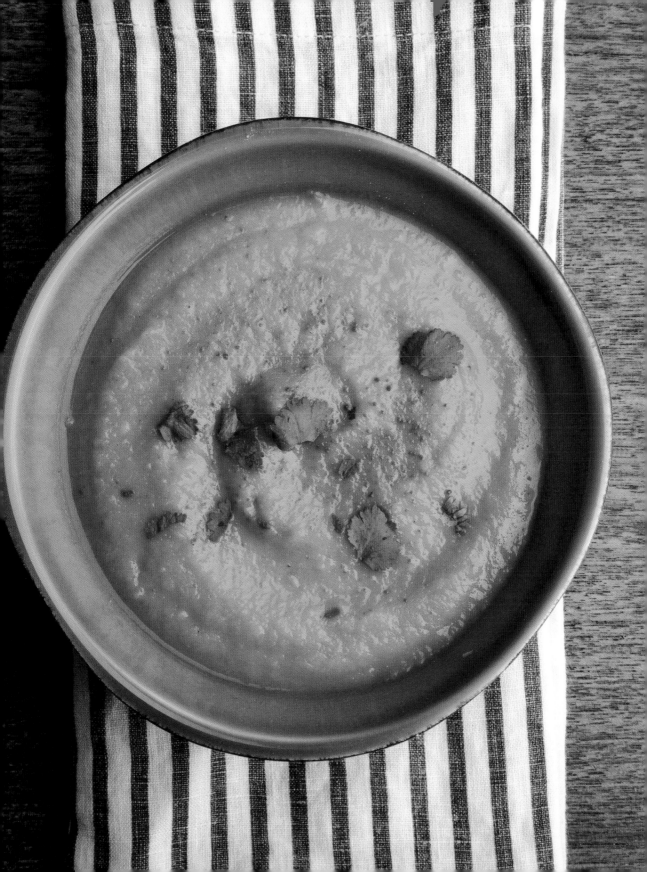

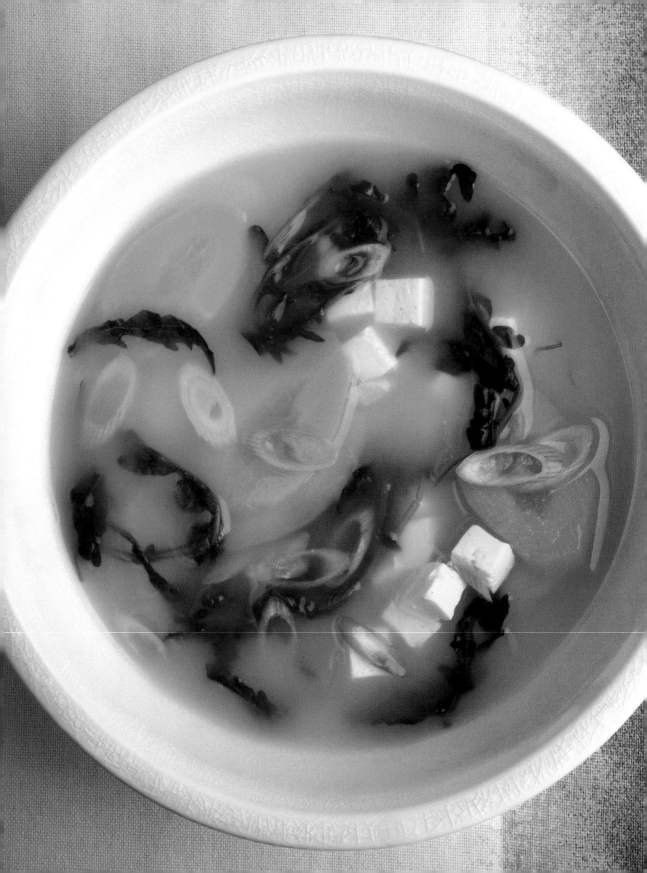

Miso Vegetable Soup with Tofu

Meal: Main, Soup

Main Ingredient:
Fermented soy

Prep Time: 15 minutes

Cook Time: 10 minutes

SERVES 2

HEALTH CONSIDERATIONS: IN TREATMENT; FATIGUE; EASY TO SWALLOW; NAUSEA; BLAND DIET; LOW FIBER; GLUTEN-FREE; HEALTHY SURVIVORSHIP; NEUTROPENIC DIET

FOOD PREFERENCE: DAIRY-FREE; VEGAN; VEGETARIAN

Miso soup is the comfort food of Japan: simple, pleasantly salty, and easy to digest. It's usually made by first making a stock, called dashi, using kombu seaweed (dried kelp). Here, instead of dashi, we use clear vegetable broth with some simple vegetables and aromatics added for flavor, some tofu for extra protein, and miso paste added at the very end. If you aren't used to cooking with miso, whisk 1 tablespoon into the soup, taste it, then add the rest 1 teaspoon at a time, tasting as you go until you get the blend that's right for you.

Health Tip

Miso is a fermented probiotic food. Many oncologists advise patients with compromised immune systems against eating live probiotics like miso or yogurt. If your doctor has advised you to stay away from probiotics but you enjoy the taste of miso, you can still eat this soup. See Ann's Tips, next page, for an easy solution.

3 cups Basic Vegetable Broth (page 21)

2 tablespoons *shiro* (white) miso (see Ann's Tips, next page)

1 small carrot, peeled and thinly sliced crosswise

2 (1-inch) slices gingerroot, julienned

2 scallions, thinly sliced crosswise

½ cup silken tofu, cut into ¼-inch dice

½ cup baby greens (spinach, arugula, or kale)

½ sheet nori seaweed, cut with scissors into thin strips

1. In a medium saucepan, bring the broth to a boil over medium-high heat. Transfer ½ cup of broth to a small bowl and whisk in the miso paste until well blended. Set aside.
2. Add the carrot and ginger to the broth and reduce the heat to medium. Cook until the carrots are just tender, about 5 minutes.
3. Add the scallions and the tofu to the broth and cook 2 minutes more to heat the tofu through. Add the baby greens and cook, covered, until greens are just wilted, about 1 minute more.
4. Turn off the heat and return the miso mixture to the saucepan. Gently stir and serve with scattered nori shreds.

Ann's Tips

· ✼ ·

Miso comes in many shades, from golden yellow to almost black. Generally speaking, the deeper the color is, the stronger the miso will taste.

Miso is a fermented, probiotic soy product. Once it is added to the soup, the soup mustn't come back to a boil or the miso will lose its live microorganisms.

If your oncologist says probiotics aren't for you, you can still enjoy this soup. Instead of stirring in the miso off the heat in step 4, add it in step 3, and simmer for 2 to 3 minutes before adding the tofu and scallions. This will make it safe, and it will still taste marvelous.

Chilled Spring Vegetable Soup

HEALTH CONSIDERATIONS: IN TREATMENT; EASY TO SWALLOW; NAUSEA; BLAND DIET; GLUTEN-FREE; NEUTROPENIC DIET; HEALTHY SURVIVORSHIP

FOOD PREFERENCE: VEGETARIAN

Meal: Main, Soup

Main Ingredients: Peas, Asparagus

Prep Time: 25 minutes

Cook Time: 45 minutes

SERVES 4 TO 6

This greenest of green soups is cool and smooth and sweetly delicious, a perfect treat to sip on if you have a sore mouth. You can add buttermilk for extra creaminess and protein, but the soup is beautifully smooth and creamy without it. I like to use chicken stock here for the extra nourishment it brings. But since the recipe makes use of the vegetable trimmings to add extra flavor, if you'd rather have a vegetarian soup, just use a clear low-sodium vegetable broth or water, making sure to add salt to taste at the end.

1 tablespoon butter

1 small leek, or 1 bunch scallions, white parts well washed and finely diced

Sea salt, to taste

1 medium Yukon Gold or white creamer potato, peeled and cut into ¼-inch dice

1 bunch thin green asparagus, cut in ¼-inch pieces, tough root ends removed

1 to 2 sprigs fresh tarragon, plus 1 tablespoon finely chopped tarragon

6 to 8 cups Basic Vegetable Broth (page 21) or Quick, Rich Chicken Broth (page 24)

1 pound frozen petite peas

½ cup buttermilk (optional)

1 tablespoon finely chopped chives

1. In a large Dutch oven, melt the butter over medium-high heat. Add the leek and sprinkle with salt, lower the heat to medium, and cook for 5 minutes, or until the leek starts to soften. Add the potato, another sprinkle of salt, and stir. Cover and cook for 5 minutes, or until the potato starts to soften. The leek should not brown, so stir the vegetables from time to time to prevent them from sticking. Add the asparagus and cook, stirring, until their color starts to brighten, about 2 minutes. Add the tarragon sprigs.

2. Pour the stock over the vegetables and bring to a boil. Once boiling, cover and

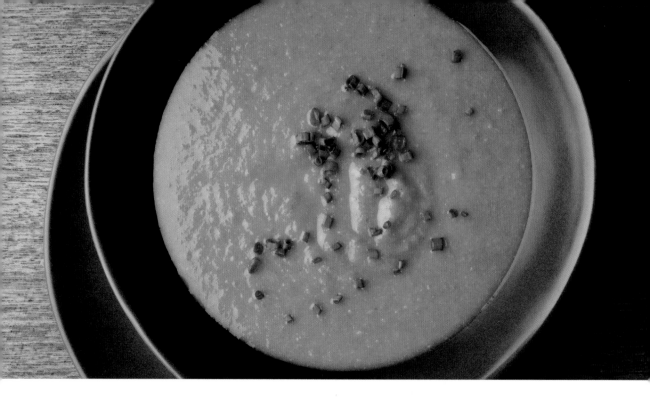

simmer for 10 minutes, or until the vegetables are tender. Add the frozen peas and cook just enough to heat them through, about 3 minutes more.

3. Blend the soup in batches or using an immersion blender until completely smooth (see page 11 for more about blending hot liquids). Check for seasoning—it's best to add extra salt while still warm. Finally, whisk in the buttermilk, if using, until blended. When cool enough, cover with a cloth and chill in the fridge. Sprinkle with chopped chives and tarragon. Serve chilled.

Ann's Tips

Leeks taste good and are very good for you, but they can be very muddy vegetables. I suggest cutting the leeks in half, placing them into a bowl of cold water, and swishing them around. Any grit or dirt will sink to the bottom, leaving the cut leeks clean.

You can save the vegetable peelings to make a batch of Basic Vegetable Broth (page 21).

Fennel Risotto

HEALTH CONSIDERATIONS: IN TREATMENT; EASY TO SWALLOW; NAUSEA; BLAND DIET; LOW FIBER; GLUTEN-FREE; NEUTROPENIC DIET

FOOD PREFERENCE: VEGETARIAN

Meal: Main

Main Ingredients: Fennel, Rice

Prep Time: 15 minutes

Cook Time: 35 minutes

SERVES 4

This is true comfort food, deliciously soothing if you're not feeling up to par, and surprisingly simple to make. Fennel is a natural digestive and, paired with white arborio rice, it is manna to a system roughed up by cancer treatment.

2 fennel bulbs with fronds

4 cups barely simmering vegetable broth (see Ann's Tips, next page)

1 tablespoon extra-virgin olive oil

1 small yellow onion, cut into small dice

Sea salt, to taste

1⅓ cups arborio rice

¼ cup dry white wine

2 tablespoons freshly grated Parmesan cheese, or to taste, plus extra for serving

2 teaspoons unsalted butter, or to taste

1. Cut the stalks and fronds off the fennel bulbs. Discard the tough stalks and reserve the feathery fronds, if there are any. Halve, quarter, and core the fennel bulbs, then cut into small dice. Roughly chop the fronds and set aside.

2. Bring the broth to a low simmer over medium-high heat. Reduce the heat to low, and keep the broth warm.

3. Heat the oil in a 5-quart Dutch oven or wok over medium-high heat. Add the diced fennel and onion and sprinkle with a little salt. Cook until the fennel is soft and the onion is translucent, about 5 minutes. Add the rice and cook, stirring until the grains start to look translucent at the edges, about 2 minutes. Add the wine and cook until it is almost all absorbed.

4. Add a ladleful of hot broth to the rice. Cook, stirring, until the rice has absorbed all the broth, 3 to 5 minutes. Add another ladleful and repeat until the rice is

just about al dente, about 20 minutes. There should be a ladleful or so of stock left.

5. Stir a ladleful of broth into the rice, this time along with 2 tablespoons of Parmesan cheese and the butter. Cook, stirring vigorously, until blended. Cover, turn off the heat, and let the rice sit for 5 minutes. Stir in the chopped fennel fronds. The risotto should be creamy looking, so if the risotto looks dry, stir in the remaining broth or some hot water, 1 tablespoon at a time, until you achieve the desired consistency. Taste for salt. Serve immediately with more Parmesan on the side.

Ann's Tips

· ✿ ·

You can also heat the stock in a microwave.

For non-vegetarians, this is extra delicious made with good chicken broth (page 24). You can also use homemade vegetable broth (page 21).

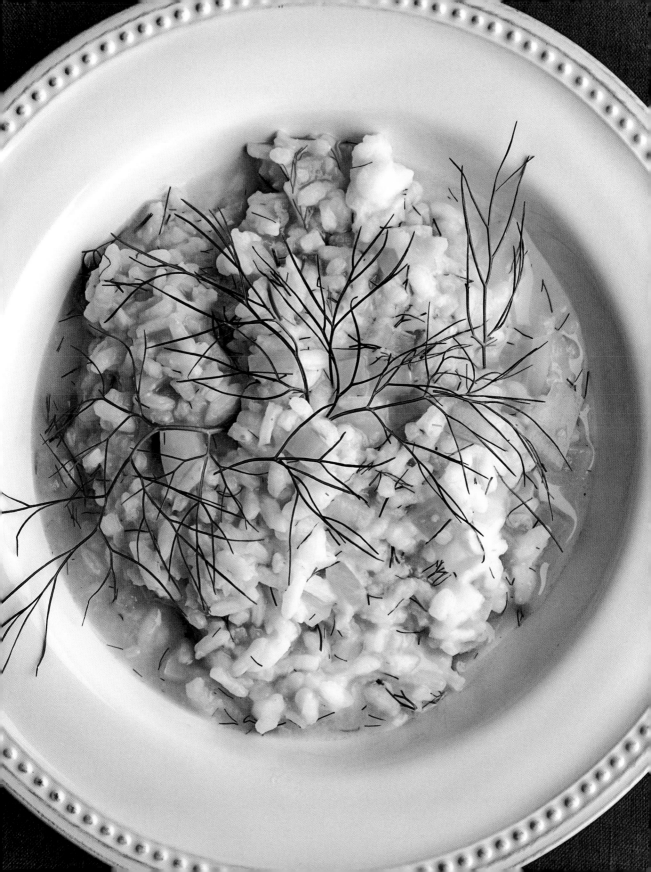

Comfy Cod and Potato Gratin

Meal: Main

Main Ingredients: Cod, Milk, Potatoes

Prep Time: 30 minutes

Cook Time: 30 minutes

SERVES 4 TO 6

HEALTH CONSIDERATIONS: IN TREATMENT; EASY TO SWALLOW; BLAND DIET; LOW FIBER; NEUTROPENIC DIET

FOOD PREFERENCE: NONE

This comforting dish is a British nursery classic. Light-tasting and delicious, it's just the kind of thing you crave when feeling poorly. The poached fish is easy to digest, and although there's some cheese, it adds subtle flavor but isn't the main event. This is easy to make, without too much prep. Just use the cooking time for the potatoes to make the sauce, and mash the potatoes while the fish is cooking. Everything will come together for baking in a jiffy.

Health Tip

If you are gluten-free, use sweet rice flour or any other GF favorite for the béchamel.

1 shallot, peeled

2 whole cloves

2 cloves garlic, peeled and smashed

1 leek, white part only, split in half and rinsed well (optional)

1 bay leaf

1 large or 2 medium Idaho potatoes (about 1 pound), cut into 1-inch dice (see Ann's Tips, next page)

Sea salt, to taste

3 tablespoons unsalted butter, divided

¼ cup grated Parmesan cheese, divided

2 tablespoons all-purpose or whole-wheat pastry flour (see Ann's Tips, next page)

1¼ cups whole or 2% milk

½ teaspoon freshly grated nutmeg

¼ cup grated Gruyère, Jarlsberg, or other mild-flavored melting cheese, divided

1½ pounds flaky mild white-flesh fish fillets such as cod, hake, or Chilean sea bass, cut into 3-inch-thick slices

1. Preheat the oven to 425°F. Grease a 2-quart baking dish and set aside.
2. Prepare the poaching liquid: Stud the shallot with the whole cloves. In a sauté pan, combine the shallot, garlic, leek (if using), bay leaf, and diced potatoes.

Sprinkle with a little salt and add just enough cold water to cover. Bring to a boil over medium-high heat. As soon as the water starts to bubble, reduce the heat to low and cook, covered, at a bare simmer for 10 minutes, or until the potatoes are soft. With a slotted spoon, transfer the potatoes to a large bowl. Reserve the liquid and aromatics in the pan and set aside. Mash the potatoes, skins and all, with ½ tablespoon of the butter and 2 tablespoons of the Parmesan cheese. Set aside.

3. While the potatoes cook, make the sauce: Melt the remaining 2½ tablespoons butter over medium-high heat in a heavy saucepan. Add the flour and cook for 1 to 2 minutes, or until you smell a slight toasty aroma. Gradually add the milk, whisking all the while. When it is all in, and the sauce has the consistency of heavy cream, add the nutmeg, the 2 tablespoons of Gruyère, and the remaining 2 tablespoons Parmesan cheese. Lower the heat to medium and cook, stirring, until the cheese has melted and the sauce begins to thicken, about 5 minutes. Taste for salt. Remove from the heat, cover, and set aside.

4. Place the fish in a single layer in the pan with the reserved liquid and aromatics. Add extra water to cover the fish if needed. Bring to a low simmer over medium heat. As soon as the water starts to bubble, reduce the heat to low and cook the fish, covered, at a bare simmer for 10 minutes. Remove the fish with a slotted spoon and transfer to a plate. Discard the cooking liquid and aromatics. Remove any skin or bones from the fish, and flake the fish with a fork.

5. Arrange the fish in the prepared baking dish. Pour the reserved sauce over the fish. Top everything with the mashed potato and sprinkle the top with the remaining 2 tablespoons Gruyère. Bake in the center of the oven until the sauce is bubbling and the top is golden in spots, about 20 minutes. Serve immediately.

Ann's Tips

·⚓·

If you are on a low-fiber diet, peel the potatoes and use all-purpose flour for the sauce.

To make the dish easier to handle and to keep your oven clean, place the baking dish on a small foil-lined baking sheet to catch drips.

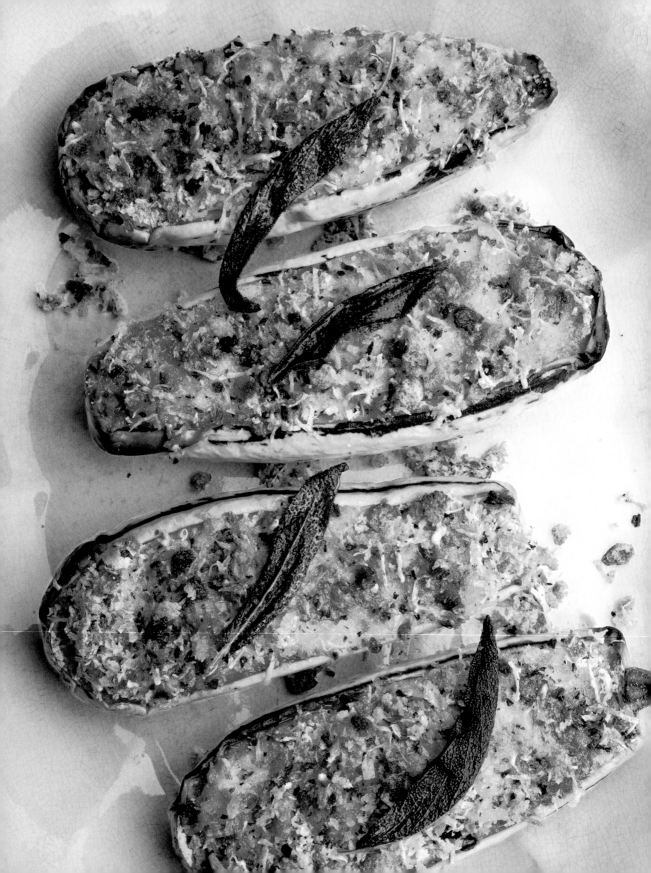

Twice-Baked Winter Squash

HEALTH CONSIDERATIONS: IN TREATMENT; FATIGUE; EASY TO SWALLOW; NAUSEA; NEUTROPENIC DIET; HEALTHY SURVIVORSHIP

FOOD PREFERENCE: VEGETARIAN

Meal: Main, Side

Main Ingredient: Winter squash

Prep Time: 20 minutes

Cook Time: 45 minutes

SERVES 4 TO 6

This is the perfect comfort food. For a delicious easy supper, squash certainly give potatoes a run for their money when cooked this way. Nutty delicata squash are my favorites. Not only does their sweet taste deepen when baked, they bring all the health benefits of winter squash to the table, notably vitamins A and C, and, since the skin is edible, fiber. Plus they are a great lower-starch substitute for other carbohydrate sources. Who could ask for anything more?

2 small to medium delicata, dumpling, or acorn squash, split in half vertically, seeds scooped out

2 cloves garlic, peeled, smashed, and minced

8 to 10 fresh sage leaves, minced, divided

Sea salt, to taste

4 teaspoons extra-virgin olive oil

½ to ¾ cup whole-wheat bread crumbs (see Ann's Tips, next page)

¼ cup freshly grated Parmesan cheese

1 cup shredded Gruyère, Jarlsberg, or mild cheddar cheese

¼ cup plain, whole milk Greek yogurt

1 teaspoon butter, or to taste

1. Preheat the oven to 400°F. Line a baking sheet with parchment paper and set aside.
2. Score the flesh of the 4 squash halves with a sharp knife. Rub in all the garlic and half the sage, and add a pinch of salt to each. Transfer to the prepared baking sheet and drizzle each half with 1 teaspoon olive oil. Bake, cut-side up, for 30 to 40 minutes, or until the flesh of the squash is soft when pierced with a fork. The cooking time will largely depend on the size of the squash. If the squash are small, test with a fork at 30 minutes.

3. As soon as the squash are soft, remove from the oven. Scoop the hot flesh into a bowl, taking care not to break the skin. Set the squash shells aside. Raise the oven temperature to broil.

4. Mix the bread crumbs, remaining sage, and Parmesan cheese together. Set aside. Mash the squash and mix in the Gruyère and the yogurt until well blended. Taste for salt. Pile the mixture back into the squash shells. Scatter the tops with the seasoned bread crumbs and dot with butter. Put under the broiler on a low shelf and cook until the tops of the squash are lightly browned, about 5 minutes. Serve immediately.

Ann's Tips

· ✈ ·

Use the smaller measure of bread crumbs if the squash are small, or don't use at all if your mouth is sore. You can make your own bread crumbs by dicing and grinding leftover bread in a food processor, and freezing what you don't use. They will keep indefinitely. This is a useful tip for thrifty cooks everywhere, including those who are gluten-free.

You can bake the squash, prepare the filling, and stuff the shells ahead of time. When you are ready to eat, add the bread crumbs and bake for 20 to 25 minutes at 375°F to heat them through, and brown the topping under the broiler.

For a more sinful version, use either mascarpone or ricotta instead of yogurt.

Steamed Vegetables and Tofu with Miso Dressing

Meal: Side

Main Ingredient: Tofu

Prep Time: 20 minutes

Cook Time: 30 minutes

SERVES 4

HEALTH CONSIDERATIONS: IN TREATMENT; FATIGUE; HIGH FIBER; GLUTEN-FREE; HEALTHY SURVIVORSHIP

FOOD PREFERENCE: DAIRY-FREE; VEGAN; VEGETARIAN; NUTS

I love simple food like this. Steaming brings out the best in vegetables while preserving their nutritional value. The sweetness of snap peas and asparagus lightly steamed with the potato and tofu is deliciously offset by a tangy white *shiro* miso dressing. A perfect easy meal.

Health Tip

Miso is a fermented probiotic food. Oncologists sometimes advise patients with compromised immune systems against eating live probiotics like miso or yogurt, so check with your doc or nurse practitioner before eating them. Miso is also high in salt, so there is no need to add any extra to the vegetables as they steam.

¾ pound sugar snap peas

6 small Yukon Gold potatoes, quartered

10 ounces firm tofu, cut into 1-inch cubes (see Ann's Tips, next page)

¾ pound green asparagus, cut into 2-inch pieces

Miso Dressing

¼ cup *shiro* (white) miso

¼ cup tahini

1 tablespoon sesame oil

1 tablespoon rice vinegar

1 tablespoon water

1. Remove and discard the stem ends and strings from the sugar snap peas.
2. Place a steamer in a pot with 1 inch of simmering water. Place the potatoes and cubed tofu in the steamer. Cover and steam for 9 minutes.
3. While the potatoes are steaming, make the dressing: In a small bowl, whisk the miso, tahini, sesame oil, vinegar, and water together. Taste, adjust seasonings, and set aside.
4. Top the potatoes with sugar snap peas and asparagus. Cover and steam for an additional 2 to 3 minutes, or until vegetables are bright green. Lift the steamer off the water and gently slide all the vegetables and tofu from the steamer onto a warm plate. Spoon the miso dressing over the vegetable mixture and serve immediately.

Ann's Tips

· ✶ ·

Many brands of tofu come in 10-ounce packages. If you can find only 16-ounce blocks, drain away the water, take what you need, and cover what's left with fresh water and some plastic wrap. It will keep for another 2 to 3 days in the fridge if you change the water daily.

If you have tree nut allergies, consider substituting sunflower seed butter for the tahini.

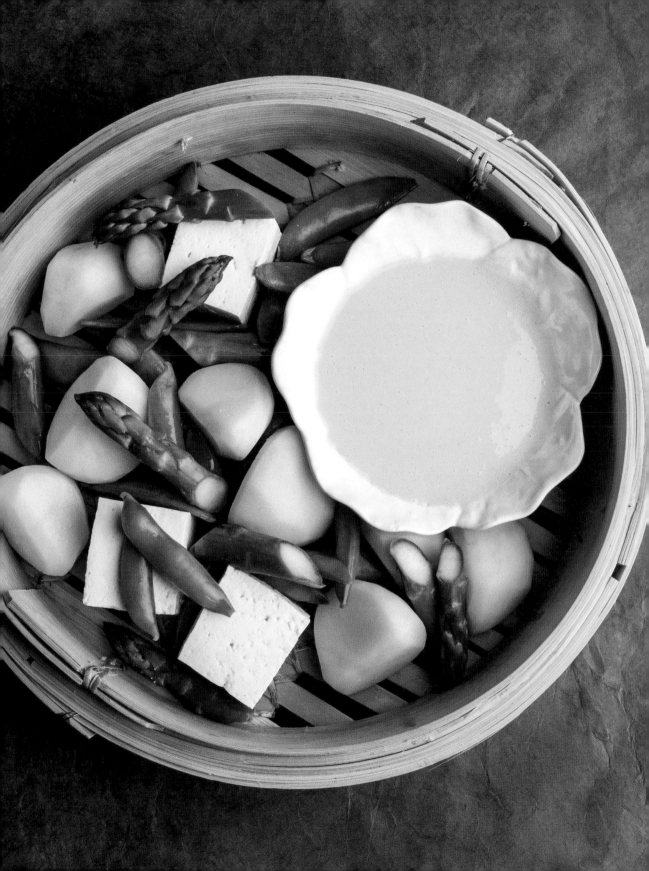

Delicious Cauliflower Puree

Meal: Side

Main Ingredient:
Cauliflower

Prep Time: 15 minutes

Cook Time: 10 minutes

SERVES 2 TO 4

HEALTH CONSIDERATIONS: IN TREATMENT; FATIGUE; EASY TO SWALLOW; NAUSEA; BLAND DIET; GLUTEN-FREE; NEUTROPENIC DIET; HEALTHY SURVIVORSHIP

FOOD PREFERENCE: VEGETARIAN (FOR VEGAN AND DAIRY-FREE, SEE ANN'S TIPS, NEXT PAGE)

This is called "delicious" because it really is delicious in its own right. Tasty and soothing to eat on its own, it makes a wonderful low-carb alternate for pureed potatoes and a perfect foil for more intensely flavored foods, such as Chicken Roasted in Cider (page 293).

1 medium head cauliflower, trimmed	1 bay leaf
1½ cups whole milk	½ teaspoon sea salt
3 cardamom pods	1 tablespoon unsalted butter (optional)

1. Break the cauliflower into medium florets.
2. Combine the milk, cardamom, bay leaf, and salt in a deep skillet or a saucepan wide enough to hold the cauliflower in one layer. Bring to a boil over medium-high heat.
3. Add the florets and reduce the heat to a simmer. Cook, partially covered, until the cauliflower is soft, about 10 minutes. The milk will be reduced by about a third. Discard the cardamom pods and bay leaf.
4. Put ½ cup of the milk in a blender. Add half of the cauliflower florets and blend until pureed. (Use caution when blending hot liquids. See page 11.) Gradually add the rest of the florets until you have a stiff yet smooth and creamy puree. Add a little more milk, 1 tablespoon at a time, if the puree is too stiff. Discard any remaining milk.

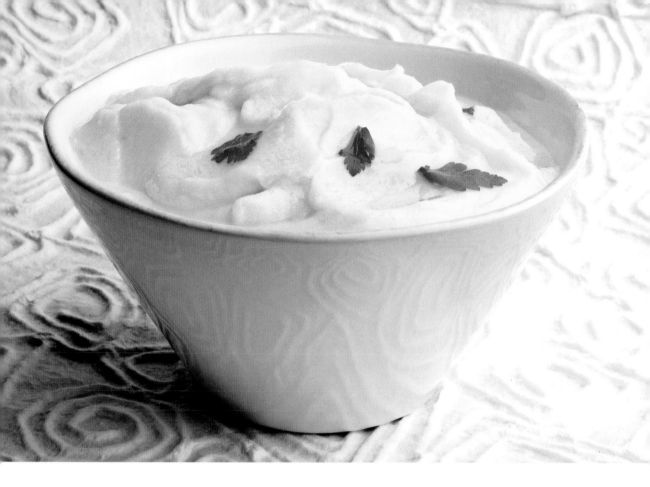

5. Return the puree to the saucepan and heat over low heat until heated through, stirring all the while. Don't let it boil. Stir in the butter, if using, and serve.

For a dairy-free vegan version, cook the cauliflower in unsweetened soy or almond milk instead of whole milk.

Ann's Tips

· ✽ ·

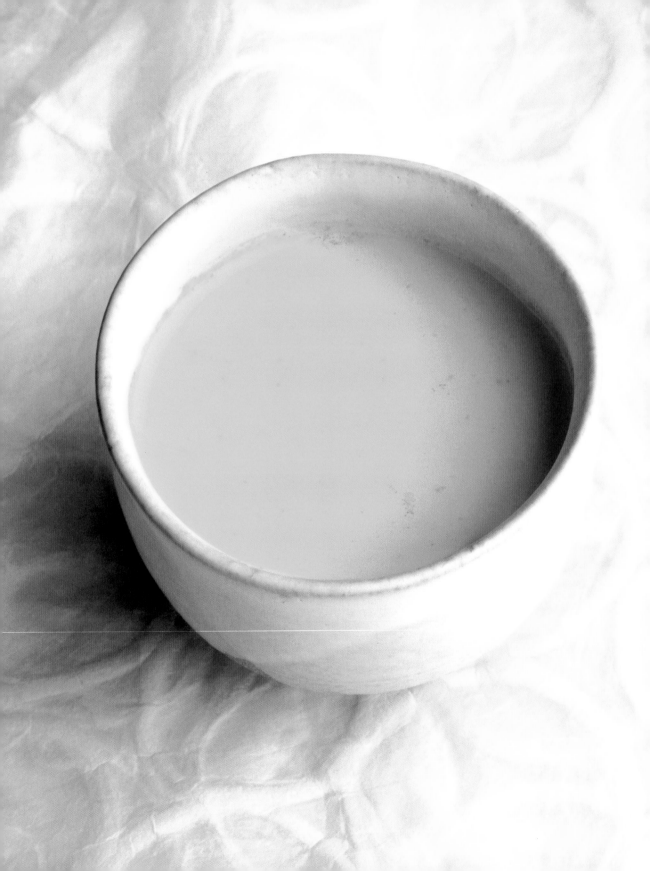

Turmeric Masala Chai Tea

HEALTH CONSIDERATIONS: IN TREATMENT; FATIGUE; EASY TO SWALLOW; NAUSEA; LOW FIBER; GLUTEN-FREE; NEUTROPENIC DIET

FOOD PREFERENCE: VEGAN; VEGETARIAN

The first time I ever had chai I was in a hole-in-the-wall Pakistani restaurant in Paris. The tea was thick, sweet and milky, and quite delicious and I have been chasing the taste ever since. This soothing drink is the closest I've come. It isn't really tea; it's more of a milky infusion using typical chai tea spices. It's one of the most comforting warm drinks you can have when you're feeling low.

Meal: Snack, Beverage

Main Ingredient: Whole milk or Non-dairy milk

Prep Time: 5 minutes

Cook Time: 10 minutes, plus 5 to 10 minutes for steeping

SERVES 1

1 cup whole or 2% milk, or unsweetened, unflavored almond or soy milk

2 green cardamom pods (see Ann's Tips, below)

¼ teaspoon freshly grated gingerroot

¼ teaspoon ground allspice, or 1 whole allspice berry

½ teaspoon ground turmeric

1 teaspoon honey or agave, to taste

1. Combine the milk, cardamom, ginger, allspice, and turmeric in a small saucepan.
2. Gradually heat over low heat until it just starts to simmer. Cook for 5 minutes, then cover and turn off the heat. Allow to steep for 5 to 10 minutes to desired strength.
3. Pour through a strainer into a ceramic cup and stir in honey to taste.

Ann's Tips

For stronger cardamom flavor, lightly crush the pods before steeping.

You can buy chai spice blends online to mix with tea. Try different blends until you find the one you like best. Most won't have turmeric, so whatever you use, add ½ teaspoon of turmeric to get the benefits of this miraculous antioxidant spice.

For extra richness, stir in 1 tablespoon of condensed milk instead of honey.

Apple-Cinnamon Oatmeal with Raisins

Meal: Breakfast

Main Ingredient: Oats

Prep Time: 10 minutes

Cook Time: 5 minutes

SERVES 4

HEALTH CONSIDERATIONS: IN TREATMENT; FATIGUE; EASY TO SWALLOW; NAUSEA; BLAND DIET; HIGH FIBER; NEUTROPENIC DIET; GLUTEN-FREE

FOOD PREFERENCE: DAIRY-FREE; VEGAN; VEGETARIAN; NUTS

Oatmeal is a classic comfort food and so easy to make. This variation is far more delicious than what comes out of a packet. You will get a whole serving of fruits, which, with the addition of protein-packed almonds, helps lower the glycemic load of the oatmeal. I've used very little added sugar, as most of the sweetness comes from the apples and raisins, but it's to taste, so you could add more. I like to make oatmeal on the stove top, since I don't like the consistency it has when microwaved. I also make it thick, the way my Scottish mother-in-law used to, so if you like your oatmeal with a lighter, creamier consistency, up the water-to-oatmeal ratio to 2¼ parts water to 1 part oatmeal; for one serving, the ratio is ¾ cup water to ⅓ cup oatmeal.

Health Tip

This is gluten-free only if you use gluten-free oats. If you have tree nut allergies, either substitute the almonds for toasted sunflower seeds or cut out the nuts altogether.

1 Gala, Fuji, or Golden Delicious apple, thinly sliced

1⅓ cups rolled oats (⅓ cup dry for 1 serving)

2⅔ cups water (⅔ cup water for 1 serving)

¼ cup golden raisins

(continued)

½ teaspoon sea salt

½ teaspoon ground cinnamon, or to taste

2 teaspoons real maple syrup, or to taste

¼ cup sliced almonds, dry-toasted (page 48)

Plain Greek yogurt or milk of your choice, to taste (optional)

1. In a medium saucepan, stir together the apple, oats, water, raisins, and salt in a pan. Bring to a boil over medium-high heat, stir well, then lower the heat to medium-low and cover. Cook for 3 to 5 minutes, or until the oatmeal has started to absorb the water and is starting to look cooked. Stir in the cinnamon and maple syrup and re-cover.

2. Cook a little longer, until the oatmeal thickens, stirring from time to time so that the oatmeal doesn't stick. Serve hot, sprinkled with the toasted almonds and a dollop of Greek yogurt, if using.

If you prefer the flavor of a tarter apple, use a Braeburn or Pink Lady apple.

Omit nuts if your mouth is sore.

Ann's Tips

· ⚓ ·

Banana-Rice Soothie

Meal: Snack, Beverage

Main Ingredients:
Banana, Cooked white rice

Prep Time: 5 minutes

Cook Time: 0 minutes

SERVES 1 TO 2

HEALTH CONSIDERATIONS: IN TREATMENT; EASY TO SWALLOW; NAUSEA; BLAND DIET; LOW FIBER; GLUTEN-FREE

FOOD PREFERENCE: DAIRY-FREE; VEGETARIAN

The name of this drink is not a typo—it's shorthand for an easy solution when you need to soothe an upset stomach or a sore mouth. This shake is intentionally very bland, so a nice ripe yellow banana with a few black spots gives the best results. If your mouth is sore from radiation, omit the vanilla.

1 ripe banana, peeled and broken into chunks

¼ cup cooked white rice

2 tablespoons whole or 2% milk or non-dairy milk

1 teaspoon honey, or to taste

½ teaspoon vanilla extract (optional)

8 ice cubes

1. Put the banana, rice, milk, honey, and vanilla, if using, into a blender along with the ice cubes. Blend until smooth.

Ann's Tips

If you keep leftover rice in the freezer, thaw before adding to the soothie.

If you have overly ripe bananas, peel them, wrap them in foil, and freeze them. They are wonderful to use as sweeteners and thickeners for shakes and smoothies. Just blend one with the milk of your choice for an easy shake.

Cozy Rice Pudding

HEALTH CONSIDERATIONS: IN TREATMENT; EASY TO SWALLOW; NAUSEA; BLAND DIET; LOW FIBER; GLUTEN-FREE; NEUTROPENIC DIET

FOOD PREFERENCE: VEGETARIAN

Meal: Dessert

Main Ingredients: Rice, Milk

Prep Time: 10 minutes

Cook Time: 45 minutes

SERVES 4

This is the perfect dish if you're going through treatment. It makes an easy, creamy rice pudding that is the ultimate comfort food when you need some TLC and don't have much energy. If you have leftover rice, even takeout rice, in your fridge or freezer, make things even simpler for yourself and use it for this deliciously satisfying dessert.

2 cups water

½ cup short-grain white rice

2¼ cups whole milk

2 tablespoons organic granulated sugar, or more to taste

⅓ cup dried fruit (raisins, dried plums, apricots, or figs)

1 teaspoon freshly grated lemon zest

Pinch of sea salt

½ teaspoon freshly grated nutmeg, or to taste

¼ cup toasted sliced almonds

Cinnamon, to taste

1. Place the water and the rice in a medium saucepan, and bring to a boil over medium-high heat. Reduce the heat to low and simmer, stirring frequently.
2. When most of the water is absorbed, 10 to 15 minutes, add the milk, sugar, and dried fruit. Simmer, stirring occasionally, for 35 to 40 minutes, or until you achieve the desired thickness.
3. Remove from the heat and stir in the lemon zest, salt, and nutmeg. Check for sweetness and add more sugar, if desired. Spoon the pudding into individual bowls, top with sliced almonds, and dust with cinnamon, if desired. Pudding can also be served cold by transferring to a glass bowl and covering with plastic wrap directly on the surface of the pudding and storing in the refrigerator.

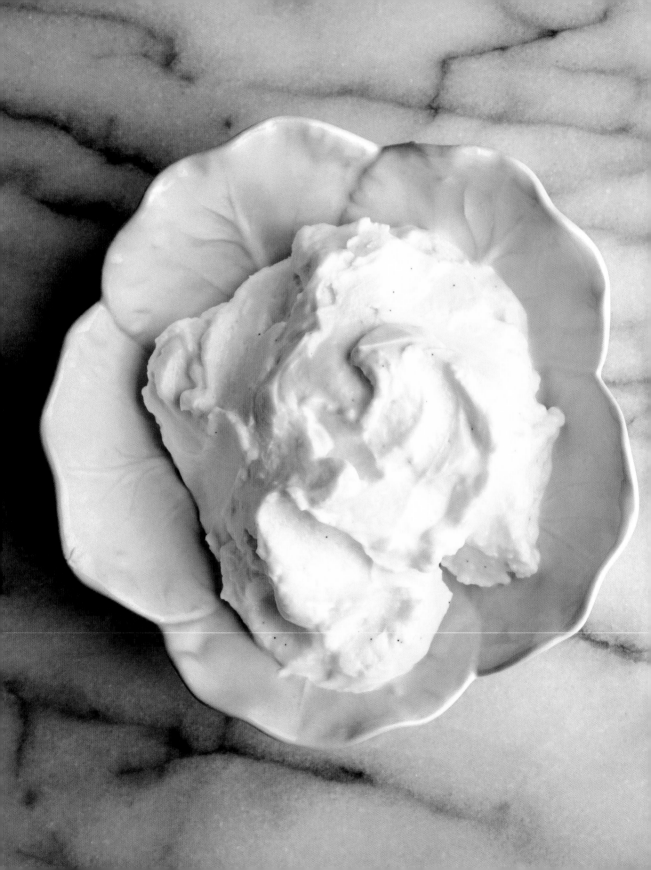

Easy Iced Treats

Creamy, cold treats are delicious anytime but can be particularly soothing to sore mouths. These easy gelatos made with creamy Greek yogurt are a firm favorite at our classes. They taste so good and are so quick to make that they offer a perfect solution when something icily sweet is in order during treatment. Here are three of our favorites. Although the methods are slightly different, the principle is always the same: either add frozen fruits to yogurt, or freeze the yogurt itself and add flavorings, which can be done even without a food processor. As you will see, it's all good, very good.

Health Tip
Yogurt is a probiotic food, so if your oncologist has warned you against eating it, sadly these treats will have to wait until your neutrophils are up. And I assure you that they are worth waiting for.

Maple Gelato

Meal: Dessert

Main Ingredient: Greek yogurt

Prep Time: 20 minutes

SERVES 4 TO 6

HEALTH CONSIDERATIONS: IN TREATMENT; EASY TO SWALLOW; FATIGUE; NAUSEA; BLAND DIET; GLUTEN-FREE; LOW FIBER

FOOD PREFERENCE: VEGETARIAN

This maple syrup–infused iced treat is a marvelously quick and great way to "à la mode" any simple dessert, plus it is cold and smooth in the mouth. You can make it ahead of time and store it in the freezer. When you're ready to eat, either let it sit in the fridge for 15 to 20 minutes to soften, or microwave for 10 seconds.

1 cup whole-milk or 2% plain Greek yogurt

⅓ cup whole or 2% milk

¼ cup maple syrup

⅛ teaspoon freshly grated nutmeg

1. Line a small, shallow baking tin or dish with parchment paper. Pile in the yogurt and smooth into a thin, even layer no more than ½ inch thick. Freeze until hard, 1½ to 2 hours depending on the thickness.
2. When you are ready for the gelato, take the frozen yogurt from the freezer and cut into smallish pieces. Put into a food processor with the milk, maple syrup, and nutmeg until a smooth soft-serve consistency is reached. Eat immediately.

Ann's Tips

· ✹ ·

Real maple syrup is the key to this simple dessert. The results just won't be the same if you use imitation syrup.

For a simpler way to make this without a food processor, check out the method for Quick Green Tea Gelato (page 137). The result will not be as light but will still be very, very good.

Quick Green Tea Gelato

HEALTH CONSIDERATIONS: IN TREATMENT; FATIGUE; EASY TO SWALLOW; NAUSEA; BLAND DIET; LOW FIBER; GLUTEN-FREE; NEUTROPENIC DIET

FOOD PREFERENCE: VEGETARIAN

Meal: Dessert

Main Ingredient: Greek yogurt, Matcha

Prep Time: 20 minutes

SERVES 4 TO 6

This easy dessert puts the antioxidants in green tea and probiotics in one treat. It's perfect for those with a mouth sore from treatment, or as a healthy(ish) sweet after a meal. Keep in mind that matcha packs quite a bit of caffeine. This dessert will not be exactly like what you'd get at a soft-serve frozen yogurt store, but for something that comes right out of your freezer with so little effort, it's a real delight.

1 cup whole-milk plain Greek yogurt

⅓ cup cold whole or 2% milk

2 tablespoons agave or honey

1 tablespoon matcha green tea powder

1. In a nonreactive bowl, mix together the yogurt, milk, agave, and matcha powder. Cover with plastic wrap and place in the freezer for 1 to 2 hours, or until completely frozen. When ready to eat, leave on the counter for 15 minutes or microwave for 20 to 30 seconds, just until it reaches an icy, creamy consistency.

You can also store the gelato in individual serving sizes so you have a quick, healthy treat anytime right out of the freezer. This also works in Popsicle molds!

Ann's Tips

· ⵙ ·

Super-Simple Gelato

Meal: Dessert

Main Ingredients: Greek yogurt, Frozen strawberries

Prep Time: 10 minutes

SERVES 6 TO 8

HEALTH CONSIDERATIONS: IN TREATMENT; FATIGUE; EASY TO SWALLOW; NAUSEA; BLAND DIET; LOW FIBER; GLUTEN-FREE

FOOD PREFERENCE: VEGETARIAN

The first time I made this gelato, I was amazed at how easy and wonderful it was. No exotic ingredients, no technique, and virtually no time are required. It's perfect for a sweet treat if you're feeling under the weather and need all the goodness fruit can bring. It's also the only way I can get my husband to eat yogurt. The main ingredients for success are frozen fruit and a food processor. Frozen fruits—and vegetables, for that matter—are picked when fully ripe and suspended in their ripeness until you're ready to use them. They are also relatively cheap, clean, and convenient to use; strawberries are already hulled, mangoes pureed or peeled and cubed, cherries pitted, and peaches sliced. Although no frozen fruits are as good as perfectly fresh ones, this recipe is a great vehicle for all of them.

1 pound frozen strawberries, or your favorite fruit

2 tablespoons water, as needed

½ cup whole-milk or 2% plain Greek yogurt

¼ cup sugar, or to taste, depending on the fruit

1. Put the strawberries into a food processor along with 1 tablespoon of the water. Pulse a couple of times, only to start breaking up the strawberries.

2. Add the yogurt and sugar. Process until just pureed and creamy, stopping to scrape down the sides of the bowl as needed. If the fruit does not break down completely, add a little more water, 1 tablespoon at a time. Take care not to over-process or your gelato will liquefy into a smoothie.

3. Serve immediately or freeze if you prefer to serve later. If frozen, allow 10 to 15 minutes for the gelato to soften at room temperature.

When using small fruits such as blueberries or cherries, or more delicate fruits such as raspberries, or frozen fruit pulp, omit step 1 and process all the ingredients together.

Greek yogurt has been strained and is very thick and creamy. The result won't be the same if you use regular plain yogurt.

Safe

· · · ✈ · · ·

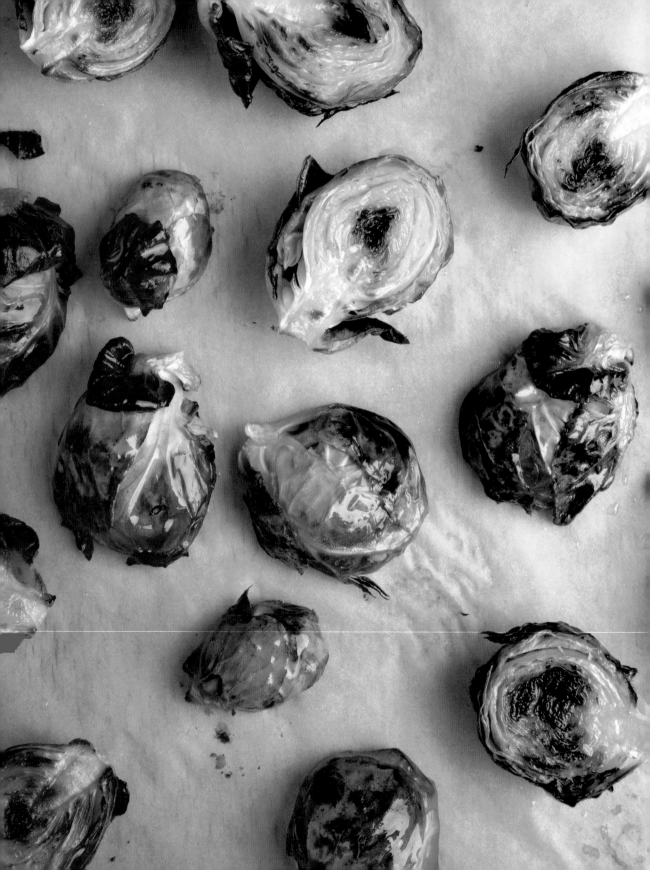

. . . . . ✈ . . . . .

During treatment, my oncologist put me on an antimicrobial diet, which meant that I could not eat any raw or undercooked foods. Not all doctors do this for all cancers, but it is a certainty that if a stem cell transplant is involved either an antimicrobial or a neutropenic diet will be part of the protocol.

This diet can feel like horrid deprivation. My doctor told me that raw fruits and berries, crunchy veggies, and salads were banned. Sushi, rare meat, and fish were off the menu, as well as certain cheeses. I was also warned to be wary of commercially prepared foods, so I couldn't rely on takeout from delis, or food from hot tables and buffets. These tough restrictions are necessary because while a healthy immune system can deal with the myriad bacteria and microbes that occur naturally on our food, these same bugs can wreak havoc on immune defenses weakened by cancer treatment.

The restrictions sink in as soon as you realize just how much the forbidden foods were part of your daily meals. I had the particular misery of being put on this diet in the summertime, so I was denied that delicious first taste of local strawberries, or the joy of biting into a juicy, ripe peach. My favorite salad greens were out of bounds, too. I wandered like a bald ghost through my favorite greenmarket, knowing that I couldn't indulge. But then I focused on what I could do to have all the forbidden things I loved: I cooked them.

I made delicious chilled salads of lightly steamed summer vegetables or roasted root vegetables dressed in tangy vinaigrettes. I enjoyed wilted greens and herbs, drizzled with a little olive oil, at room temperature. I made compotes from soft summer fruits, which I chilled and ate on their own or froze into granitas or gelatos. No deprivation there. The moral of this story? If you can't make lemons into lemonade, make cherries into compote. Here are some tasty ideas to get you safely and deliciously through your treatment.

SAFE RAW FRUITS

The insides of thick-skinned fruits like melons are sterile. If their outer skins are thoroughly washed before you cut into them, their insides can be eaten with impunity. This allows watermelon, cantaloupe, and honeydews; avocados; and, of course, citrus fruits back into the mix. Try experimenting with the more exotic thick-skinned tropical fruits, too. All are extremely nutritious. I'm now a huge fan of mangoes, papayas, and even the unusual-looking dragon fruit.

USING FRESH HERBS

In my recipes, I often suggest adding fresh herbs at the end of cooking, to boost flavor. If you are on a neutropenic or antimicrobial diet, you can still do this, but to be safe you must continue the cooking for at least 3 minutes after adding them to the dish.

PROBIOTICS

If you are following a neutropenic diet, check with your doctor or registered dietitian to determine if yogurt, miso, kimchi, and other probiotic foods are within your dietary guidelines. It's important to ask. Some medical centers recommend that immunocompromised patients avoid the probiotics in yogurt, while others feel that these healthy bacteria may be particularly beneficial to someone with a weak immune system.

Tomato Upside-Down Cake

HEALTH CONSIDERATIONS: GLUTEN-FREE; IN TREATMENT; HIGH FIBER; HEALTHY SURVIVORSHIP; NEUTROPENIC DIET

FOOD PREFERENCE: DAIRY-FREE; VEGAN; VEGETARIAN

Meal: Main

Main Ingredients:
Chickpea flour, Tomatoes

Prep Time: 30 minutes

Cook Time: 50 minutes

MAKES 1 (9-INCH) CAKE

This savory, summery, Mediterranean-style vegan treat is as delicious as it is nutritious. It is basically a healthy tomato tarte tatin, and a total taste treat. Instead of puff pastry, the roasted tomatoes are covered by a rich moist *farinata*. Tomatoes are full of the cancer-protective anti-oxidant lycopene, which becomes more accessible to our bodies when tomatoes are cooked, while the protein-packed *farinata* batter is made with mineral-rich garbanzo flour, monounsaturated olive oil, and nutritious silken tofu. Bottom line: It's not only really good to eat, it's really, really good for you.

½ cup extra-virgin olive oil, divided

10 to 12 ripe plum tomatoes, halved and seeds gently squeezed out

4 shallots, halved

8 to 10 oil-cured black olives (optional), pitted and halved

3 sprigs thyme, leaves stripped

½ teaspoon sea salt, plus more to taste

½ cup silken tofu

1 cup chickpea flour

1 teaspoon baking powder

½ teaspoon smoked sweet paprika

1¼ cups cold water, divided (see Ann's Tips, next page)

1. Preheat the oven to 400°F. Line a baking sheet with parchment and set aside. You will also need a 9-inch cast-iron skillet or round cake pan (not springform).
2. Put 1 tablespoon of the olive oil into a large bowl. Add the tomatoes, gently tossing to coat well, then transfer them to the prepared baking sheet in a single layer. Repeat with the shallots, adding a little more oil if needed. Place the baking sheet on a rack in the upper third of the oven for 15 to 20 minutes, or until the tomatoes are softened and have given up some of their liquid and the shal-

lots have started to color. Remove from the oven and set aside. Reduce the oven temperature to 375°F.

3. Add 1 tablespoon of the oil to the skillet. If using a cake pan, line the bottom with a circle of parchment paper. Add the tomato halves skin-side down in one tight layer, tucking in the shallots, and sprinkle with the olives (if using), the thyme leaves, and salt. Place the pan on a rack set in middle third of oven while you make the batter.

4. Meanwhile, in a blender, combine ⅓ cup of the olive oil and the tofu. Blend until smooth. Set aside. Sift the chickpea flour, baking powder, ½ teaspoon of salt, and paprika into a large mixing bowl. Make a well in the flour mixture and stir in the contents of the blender, scraping down the sides of the bowl as you go. Gradually whisk the batter together, making sure there are no lumps. (You can also use a hand mixer to do this.) Beat in the water, ¼ cup at a time, using just enough to make a smooth batter the consistency of heavy cream.

5. Take the hot skillet out of the oven and gently pour the batter over the roasted tomatoes. Drizzle any remaining olive oil over the top. Return to the oven. Bake for 45 to 50 minutes or until light golden and a skewer inserted in the center of the cake comes out clean. Let cool in the skillet on a wire rack for 15 minutes to finish cooking.

6. To turn out: Run a thin metal spatula around the edge of the pan. Place a plate on top, then turn the whole thing over. Lift the pan off. Serve warm or at room temperature with a salad of crisp greens.

Ann's Tips

· ✚ ·

When you put the tofu mixture into the bowl, blend the first ¼ cup of water you plan to use for the batter in the dirty blender. It will not only get any remaining batter off, but also clean your blender blades!

If you are not strictly vegan, try adding ¼ cup of shaved Parmesan cheese on top of the tomatoes before adding the batter.

If you use olives, go easy on the salt in step 3.

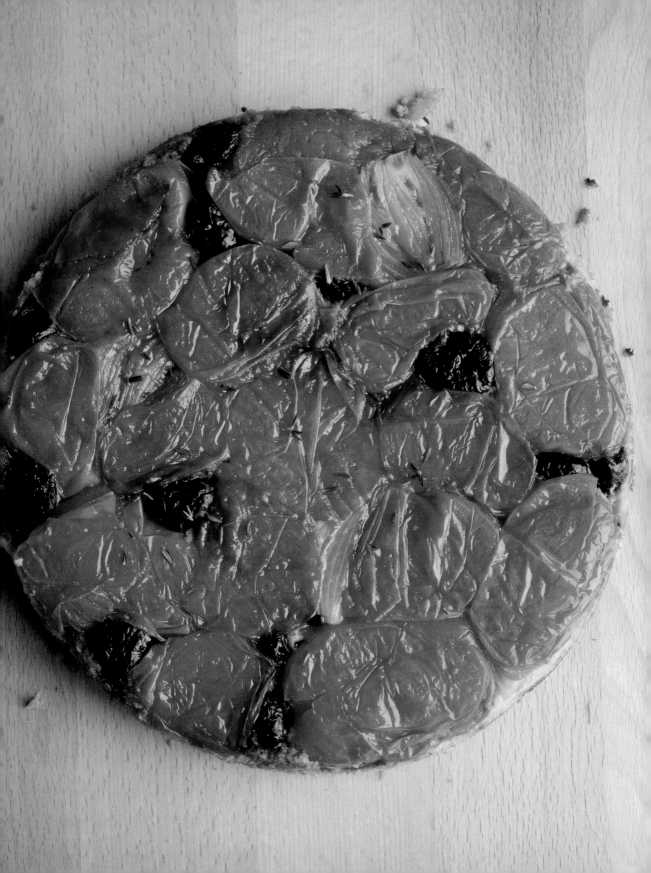

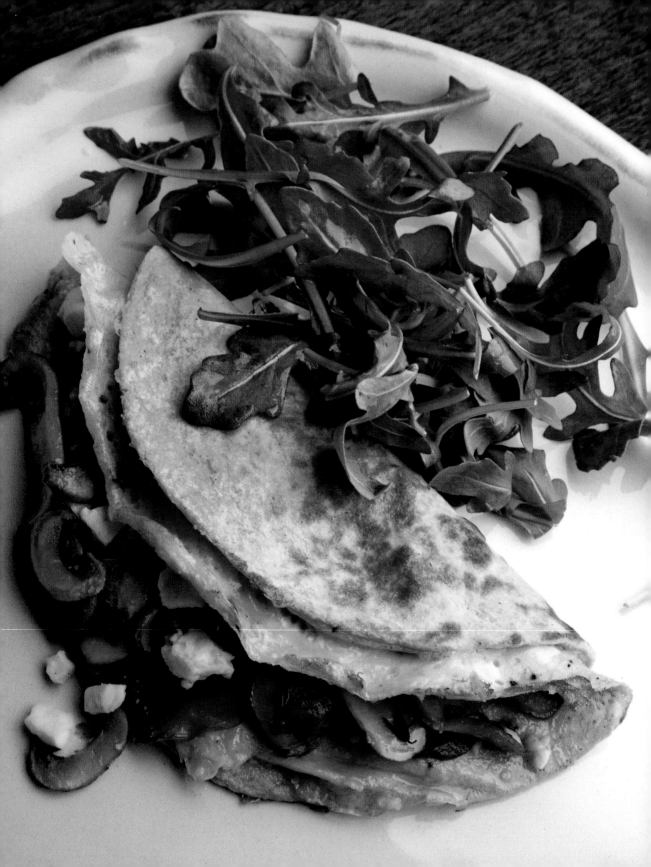

Egg Quesadilla with Sautéed Mushrooms

HEALTH CONSIDERATIONS: IN TREATMENT; FATIGUE; GLUTEN-FREE; NEUTROPENIC DIET

FOOD PREFERENCE: VEGETARIAN

Meal: Main

Main Ingredients: Eggs, Mushrooms

Prep Time: 10 minutes

Cook Time: 15 minutes

MAKES 2 (6-INCH) QUESADILLAS

Quesadillas are great standbys for quick lunches or snacks. They can also make great breakfasts. This fabulously tasty version is a treat for those in treatment. The spicy mushrooms are just heavenly, and I love how it uses one pan to cook the eggs and warm the tortilla at the same time. Once you flip them over and have spooned on the mushrooms and feta, you're all set.

2 large eggs

Sea salt and freshly ground black pepper, to taste

4 large white button mushrooms, stems removed and tops wiped clean with damp paper towel

1 tablespoon extra-virgin olive oil, divided

1 small shallot, peeled and thinly sliced

1 sprig thyme, leaves stripped and chopped

Pinch of smoked paprika

2 teaspoons Worcestershire sauce

2 (6-inch) corn tortillas

2 tablespoons crumbled feta cheese, divided

1. In a bowl, beat the eggs with a pinch of salt and some freshly ground pepper. Set aside. Thickly slice the mushroom tops. Set aside.
2. In a small skillet, heat 2 teaspoons of the olive oil over medium-high heat. Add the shallot and thyme and cook until the shallot has wilted and started to color, about 3 minutes. Add the mushrooms and sprinkle with salt and the smoked paprika. Cook, stirring, until the mushrooms wilt and give up some of their

juices and have darkened. Add the Worcestershire sauce and cook 1 minute more. Cover and remove from the heat while you make the quesadillas.

3. In another small skillet, heat half the remaining olive oil over medium heat. Pour in half the beaten egg, let cook for about 20 seconds, then top with 1 corn tortilla. Once the egg has set, after about 1 minute, flip so the tortilla is on the bottom. Scatter half the feta cheese over the egg and spoon half the reserved mushrooms on top. Fold over and hold closed for a few seconds, then transfer to a plate. Repeat with the remaining egg, tortilla, and mushroom mixture. Serve immediately.

Ann's Tips

·⚓·

On their own, the mushrooms in this recipe make a great snack over a slice of buttered multigrain toast. And try other fillings for this eggy tortilla, like sliced avocado and a little salsa, as long as it's the jarred and pasteurized variety. It's also a great way to repurpose leftovers, like topping the eggs with Smoky Black Bean Chili with Farro (page 197).

Savory Polenta Bowl with Egg, Sun-Dried Tomatoes, and Feta

HEALTH CONSIDERATIONS: IN TREATMENT; FATIGUE; EASY TO SWALLOW; NAUSEA; GLUTEN-FREE; NEUTROPENIC DIET

FOOD PREFERENCE: VEGETARIAN

Meal: Breakfast, Main

Main Ingredients: Polenta, Eggs

Prep Time: 15 minutes

Cook Time: 20 minutes

SERVES 2

Polenta is where the comfort food of Italy meets the American South. Polenta is basically yellow cornmeal grits. Luckily for us, like grits, quick-cooking versions of polenta are almost easier to find than the slow-cooking originals, which makes this dish a snap for a tasty, hearty, healthy breakfast. Sun-dried tomatoes and a sprinkle of fresh thyme take the taste place of bacon, while soft-boiled eggs replace fried eggs. A drizzle of a little good heart-healthy olive oil completes the dish. Hardly deprivation.

Health Tip

An important note about eating eggs during treatment: Because of occasional issues with salmonella in raw eggs, to be on the safe side, always cook eggs until the yolks are completely cooked. This will deal with unwanted microbes that can have a stronger effect when your immune system is compromised.

1½ cups water or Basic Vegetable Broth (page 21)

Sea salt, to taste

½ cup yellow cornmeal, instant polenta, or quick-cooking grits

1 tablespoon extra-virgin olive oil or butter

1 tablespoon grated Parmesan cheese

2 Soft- or Hard-Boiled Eggs (page 29)

(continued)

2 tablespoons chopped dehydrated sun-dried tomatoes (see Ann's Tips, below)

¼ cup crumbled feta cheese

1 teaspoon fresh thyme leaves

Freshly ground black pepper, to taste

1. In a medium, heavy saucepan, bring the water and salt to a boil. Gradually whisk in the cornmeal, stirring constantly. Reduce the heat to low and continue to stir for about 5 minutes. Stir in the olive oil and Parmesan cheese. Turn off the heat, cover, and allow the polenta to sit for 5 minutes.

2. Divide the polenta between 2 bowls, top each with an egg and an equal amount of chopped sun-dried tomato, feta cheese, thyme, a drizzle of good olive oil, and black pepper.

Ann's
Tips
· ✦ ·

Buy prepackaged sun-dried tomatoes, as those from the bulk section are not safe for patients following a neutropenic diet.

If the sun-dried tomatoes are hard, soak in hot water for 20 minutes to soften.

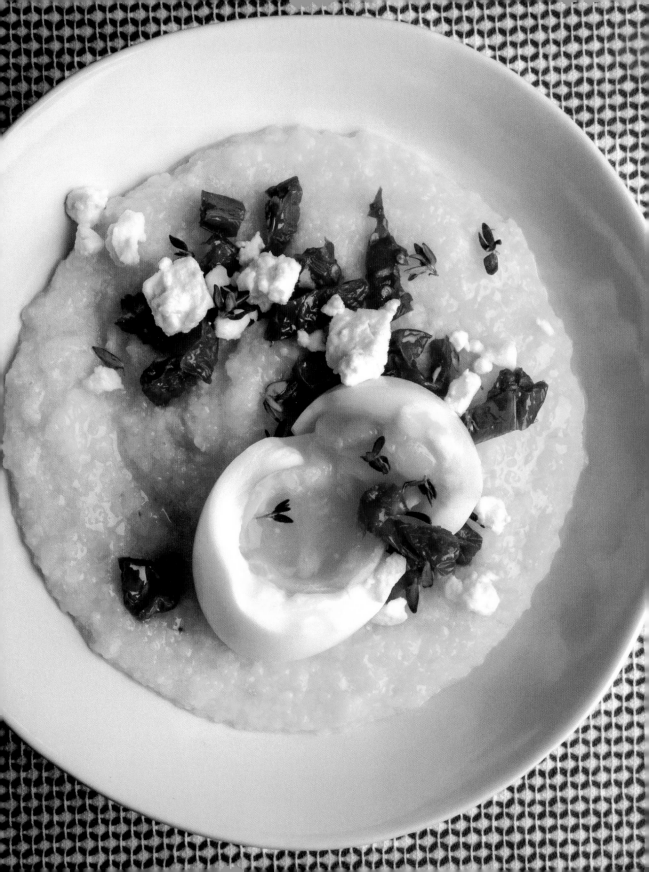

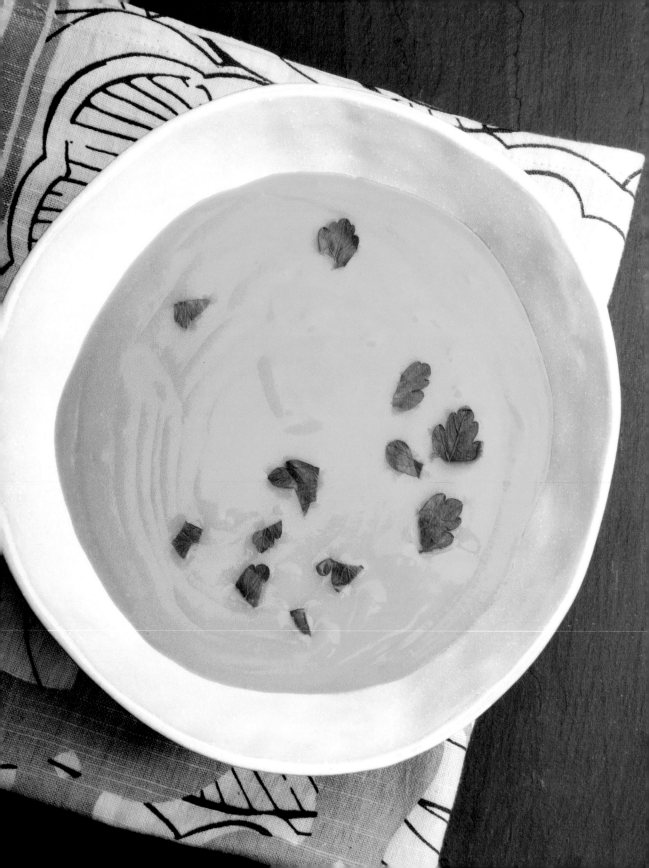

Creamy Winter Squash Soup

HEALTH CONSIDERATIONS: GLUTEN-FREE; BLAND DIET; IN TREATMENT; LOW FIBER; EASY TO SWALLOW; HEALTHY SURVIVORSHIP; NAUSEA; FATIGUE; NEUTROPENIC DIET

FOOD PREFERENCE: VEGETARIAN

Meal: Main, Soup

Main Ingredients: Winter squash, Fennel

Prep Time: 20 minutes

Cook Time: 35 minutes

SERVES 4 TO 6

This soup goes fast. Kabocha has a soft, starchy consistency and a quite wonderful nutty flavor that works great with potatoes. Cutting the kabocha is the most intensive thing you have to do for this recipe, but easy does it. If your energy's low and your local store has precut butternut squash, go for that instead. The soup may turn out a little less creamy but will still be delicious and soothing.

Health Tip

If you are struggling with nausea or need to follow a particularly bland diet, you can leave out some of the stronger flavors in this recipe, such as the onion and paprika, for a very simple, nourishing, and comforting soup.

2 tablespoons extra-virgin olive oil

1 medium onion, diced (see Ann's Tips, next page)

½ fennel bulb, diced

1 bay leaf

Sea salt, to taste

1 small kabocha or butternut squash, peeled, seeded, and cut into 1-inch dice

1 medium Yukon Gold potato, scrubbed and cut into medium dice

1 teaspoon sweet paprika

⅓ cup whole milk or 2% plain Greek yogurt

6 cups low-sodium Basic Vegetable Broth (page 21), Quick, Rich Chicken Broth (page 24), or water

2 teaspoons unsalted butter (optional)

Chopped fresh flat-leaf parsley, for garnish

1. Heat the oil in a Dutch oven over medium-high heat. Add the onion, fennel, and bay leaf. Cook for 1 minute. Sprinkle with salt, reduce the heat to medium, and gently sauté the vegetables for 5 minutes. Add the squash and potato, sprinkle with a little more salt, and stir to mix. Gently cook for 15 minutes more, stirring from time to time, until the vegetables have started to soften.

2. Increase the heat to medium-high and sprinkle the paprika over the vegetables. Cook, stirring, for 1 minute, then stir in the yogurt. Increase the heat to high.

3. Cook, stirring, until all the liquid in the yogurt boils away. Add the stock and bring to a boil. Cover and reduce the heat to a simmer. Cook until you can smash the squash and potato against the sides of the pan, 10 to 15 minutes more.

4. Transfer the soup in batches to a blender and blend at high speed until smooth. (Use caution when blending hot liquids. See page 11.) Return the soup to the pan and bring to a simmer. Stir in the butter, if using. Let the soup sit for 5 minutes. Sprinkle with parsley and serve.

Ann's Tips

· ⊤ ·

If kabocha winter squash (also sold as calabasa squash) is hard to come by in your area, delicata has a similar mealy texture, but that great kitchen all-rounder butternut squash will do the job perfectly well. With butternut, I would use a medium Idaho baking potato, peeled and diced, instead of Yukon Gold, as its super-starchy texture will make up for the creaminess the butternut lacks.

If you are on a neutropenic diet, cook the parsley garnish in the soup for 3 minutes.

Creamy Mushroom Soup

HEALTH CONSIDERATIONS: IN TREATMENT; EASY TO SWALLOW; NEUTROPENIC DIET; HEALTHY SURVIVORSHIP

FOOD PREFERENCE: DAIRY-FREE; VEGAN; VEGETARIAN

Meal: Soup

Main Ingredients: Mushrooms, Farro

Prep Time: 30 minutes

Cook Time: 50 minutes

SERVES 4 TO 6

Mushrooms are so good for you—and tasty, too! They are bursting with vitamins and minerals. Asian mushrooms, such as shiitake and maitake, have recently become popular for their immune-boosting effects, as well as possibly reducing side effects of cancer treatment. This smooth, thick, satisfying soup is easy, delicious, and dairy-free. The soaking water from the dried mushrooms is full of flavor and helps to make a great broth, while farro is a deliciously nutritious update on the more usual barley. Give it a try.

½ ounce dried porcini or shiitake mushrooms (see Ann's Tips, next page)

1 cup hot water

1 medium portobello mushroom, trimmed and wiped clean with damp paper towel

2 cups (about 8 ounces) white button mushrooms, trimmed and wiped clean with damp paper towel

2 tablespoons extra-virgin olive oil, plus extra for drizzling

3 medium shallots, peeled and minced

2 sprigs fresh thyme, leaves stripped and chopped

2 cloves garlic, minced

1 teaspoon sea salt, or to taste

¼ teaspoon smoked paprika

½ cup farro

4 cups Basic Vegetable Broth (page 21) or water (see Ann's Tips, next page)

1 tablespoon unsalted butter (optional)

Greek yogurt, for garnish (optional)

1. Cover the dried mushrooms with the hot water. Cover and let soak for 15 minutes.
2. Meanwhile, dice the portobello mushroom and quarter the button mushrooms.

Set aside. Drain the soaked mushrooms, reserving the soaking liquid. Chop the soaked mushrooms and strain the soaking liquid into a bowl. Set both aside.

3. Heat the oil in a Dutch oven over medium heat. Add the shallots, thyme, and garlic. Sprinkle with a little of the salt and the smoked paprika. Cook, stirring, until the shallots start to take on color, about 5 minutes. Add the mushrooms and sprinkle with a little more salt. Raise the heat to medium-high. Cook, stirring occasionally, until the mushrooms have wilted and browned and given up their juices, 10 to 15 minutes.

4. Add the farro and stir to mix. Add the mushroom soaking liquid and vegetable broth. Bring the mixture to a boil, then reduce the heat to medium-low. Simmer for 30 to 40 minutes, or until the farro is tender.

5. Blend the soup in batches in a blender until smooth and creamy. (Use caution when blending hot liquids. See page 11.) Taste for salt. Return the soup to the Dutch oven and heat through and stir in the butter, if using. Serve drizzled with olive oil and topped with a dollop of Greek yogurt, if desired.

Ann's
Tips

· ✈ ·

If you aren't strictly vegetarian, you can use chicken broth (page 24). If you opt to use water instead of broth or stock, you may need to add more salt at the end of cooking.

If you can't find farro, use either spelt or hulled barley. You may need to add an extra 10 minutes to the cooking time if you do.

Dried shiitake mushrooms have hard, woody stems. After soaking, cut away the tough stems and discard before using the mushrooms.

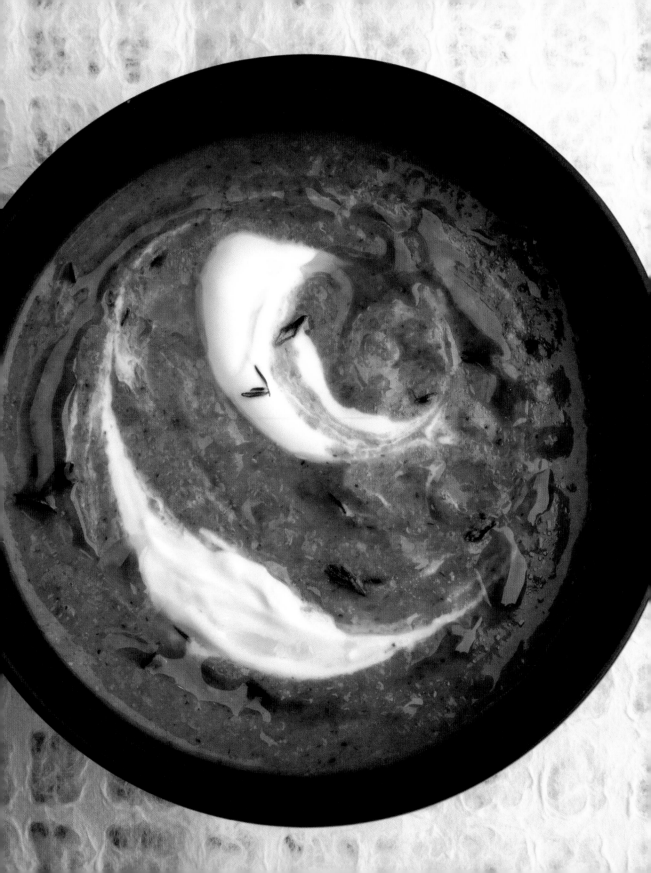

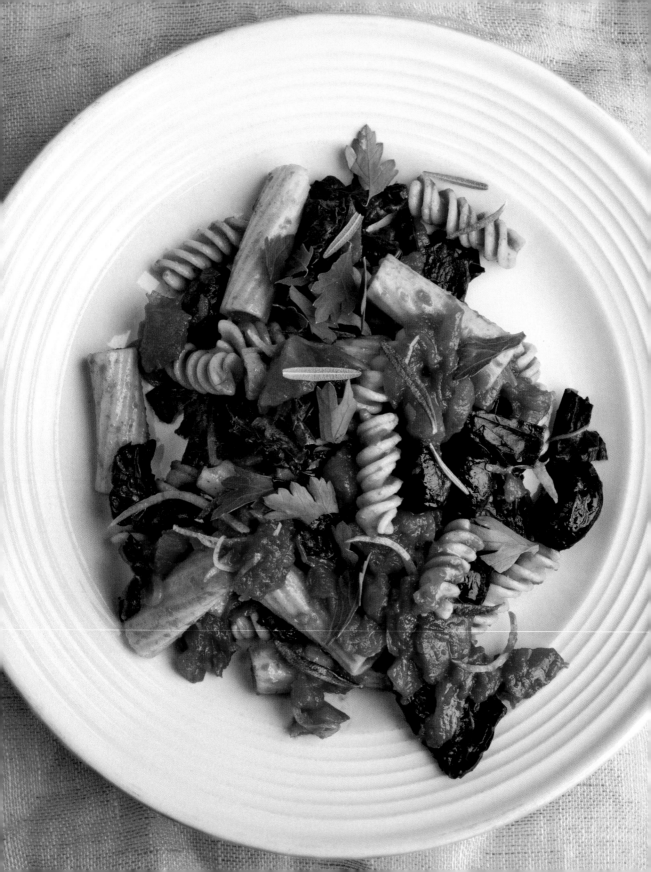

Pasta with Kale and Black Olives

Meal: Main

Main Ingredients: Kale, Whole-wheat pasta

Prep Time: 15 to 20 minutes

Cook Time: 25 minutes

SERVES 4

HEALTH CONSIDERATIONS: IN TREATMENT; HEALTHY SURVIVORSHIP; HIGH FIBER; NEUTROPENIC DIET

FOOD PREFERENCE: VEGETARIAN

This recipe is super fast, super easy, and super tasty. You can have it on the table in the time it takes the pasta to cook. I happen to prefer whole canned tomatoes, but if you'd rather not have the extra work, diced will do the job. Same thing goes for the kale; don't hesitate to use precut, or, for even less work, frozen. Frozen kale can simply be added at the end of step 3.

3 quarts water

1 tablespoon sea salt, plus more to taste

8 ounces whole-wheat penne or rigatoni

2 tablespoons extra-virgin olive oil

3 cloves garlic, smashed and sliced

1 whole dried cayenne pepper (optional)

1 medium shallot, peeled and thinly sliced

½ teaspoon sweet smoked paprika

1 (2-inch) strip lemon zest, julienned

1 (10-ounce) box frozen kale or 1 bunch lacinato or dinosaur kale, steamed (see Ann's Tips, next page)

1 (14-ounce) can diced tomatoes, chopped (see Ann's Tips, next page)

10 to 12 oil-cured black olives

2 tablespoons freshly grated Parmesan cheese, plus more for serving

½ cup flat-leaf parsley, chopped

1 small sprig rosemary, leaves stripped and chopped

Freshly ground black pepper, to taste

1. Combine the water and salt and bring to a boil.
2. Add the pasta to the boiling water. Cook for 1 minute less than the time indicated on the package instructions, approximately 10 minutes. When the pasta is

ready, drain, reserving 1 cup of the cooking water. Set aside. (See Ann's Tips, below.)

3. Meanwhile, heat the oil in a sauté pan over medium-high heat. Add the garlic and dried cayenne pepper, if using, and cook until the garlic starts to turn light golden, about 2 minutes. Add the shallot, sprinkle with salt, and cook the shallot until it softens and starts to color, about 5 minutes. Add the paprika and lemon zest, stir to coat, then add the kale and cook, stirring, until well mixed.

4. Add the tomatoes and the olives. Cook over medium heat until the tomatoes look orangey and saucy, 5 to 7 minutes. Add ½ cup of the reserved pasta cooking water and stir to mix. Add the Parmesan cheese. Cook, stirring, until it melts into the sauce and the extra water has almost evaporated, about 2 minutes. Do not add salt without tasting—the olives will have added quite a bit.

5. Stir in the parsley and rosemary. Add the cooked pasta and ¼ cup more of the reserved pasta cooking water. Cook, stirring, until the pasta is just al dente, adding more of the reserved water if the pasta looks dry. Serve immediately with a grind or two of black pepper and some freshly grated Parmesan cheese.

Ann's Tips

If you can't find lacinato, or dinosaur, kale, use regular curly kale prepped as in Steaming and Freezing Greens at Home (page 36).

In the summertime, when tomatoes are good, use 2 cups chopped ripe beefsteak or Roma tomatoes.

Spanish-Style Cod with Chickpeas and Peppers

HEALTH CONSIDERATIONS: IN TREATMENT; FATIGUE; GLUTEN-FREE; NEUTROPENIC DIET; HEALTHY SURVIVORSHIP

FOOD PREFERENCE: DAIRY-FREE

Meal: Main
Main Ingredient: Fish
Prep Time: 25 minutes, plus 30 minutes for marinating
Cook Time: 40 minutes
SERVES 6

I love the cuisine of Spain. Spanish cooking has its roots in Morocco, and thanks to the roving Spaniards who came to the New World to find riches, elements of this way of cooking have found their way all over the Americas. From Chile to Mexico to the Caribbean to Florida and points north, you can find Spanish influence in cuisine. This hearty, nutritious dish can be ready for the table in about an hour. It is based on a traditional fish stew made with *bacalao*, or salt cod, a staple of this roving cuisine. The long soaking time that salt cod needs turns what is basically a very tasty, very quick dish into a time-consuming one—not something I'd recommend when energy is at a premium. Luckily, fresh cod, though milder in taste, works just as well, and in partnership with the distinctive flavor of smoked paprika gives us an easy, delicious one-pot meal.

1 (2½-pound) cod fillet, cut into 6 pieces

2 teaspoons ground cumin

Juice of 1 lemon, divided

Pinch of saffron threads (optional)

¼ cup boiling water

2 tablespoons extra-virgin olive oil

1 teaspoon cumin seeds

3 cloves garlic, smashed and sliced

1 large Spanish onion, halved and thinly sliced

3 red peppers, deseeded and thinly sliced

2 bay leaves

Sea salt, to taste

1 teaspoon smoked paprika (see Ann's tips, next page)

1 (14-ounce) can diced tomatoes

1 (14-ounce) can chickpeas, rinsed and drained

1. Pat the fish dry and rub with the ground cumin. Place in a large bowl with half the lemon juice. Mix well and marinate in the fridge for 30 minutes.
2. Soak the saffron threads in the boiling water, if using. Set aside.
3. Heat the oil in a large sauté pan over medium heat. Add the cumin seeds, let them sizzle for a few minutes until they become fragrant, then add the garlic and cook until it starts to color, about 1 minute. Add the onion, peppers, and bay leaves. Sauté until the vegetables start to soften, 3 to 5 minutes. Sprinkle with salt, cover, and reduce the heat to medium-low. Cook gently for 10 minutes, stirring from time to time, or until the vegetables are soft and the onions are a pale gold.
4. Increase the heat to medium-high. Sprinkle the vegetables with the paprika and cook, stirring, for 1 minute. Add the tomatoes and soaked saffron and its water. Cook until the tomatoes have lost most of their liquid. Add the chickpeas and cook until heated through, 5 to 8 minutes. You can prepare the dish ahead of time up to this point.
5. Lay the fish on top of the vegetables. Cover. Bring to a boil, then reduce the heat and simmer for 5 minutes.
6. Add the remaining lemon juice. Cover and cook 2 minutes more, turn off the heat, and allow the fish to steam for 5 to 10 minutes. Serve immediately.

Ann's Tips

When buying the cod fillet, ask the fishmonger to cut your fish from the thicker head end of the fillet so that it is of even thickness and cooks at the same speed. He can also slice it for you.

The flavor of smoked paprika is a major element of this dish. Don't substitute any other kind.

Saffron has to be hand harvested and, as a result, both the threads and powder are very expensive. It gives wonderful flavor to fish stews like this one, so if you can spring for it, do so, knowing that a little goes a long way.

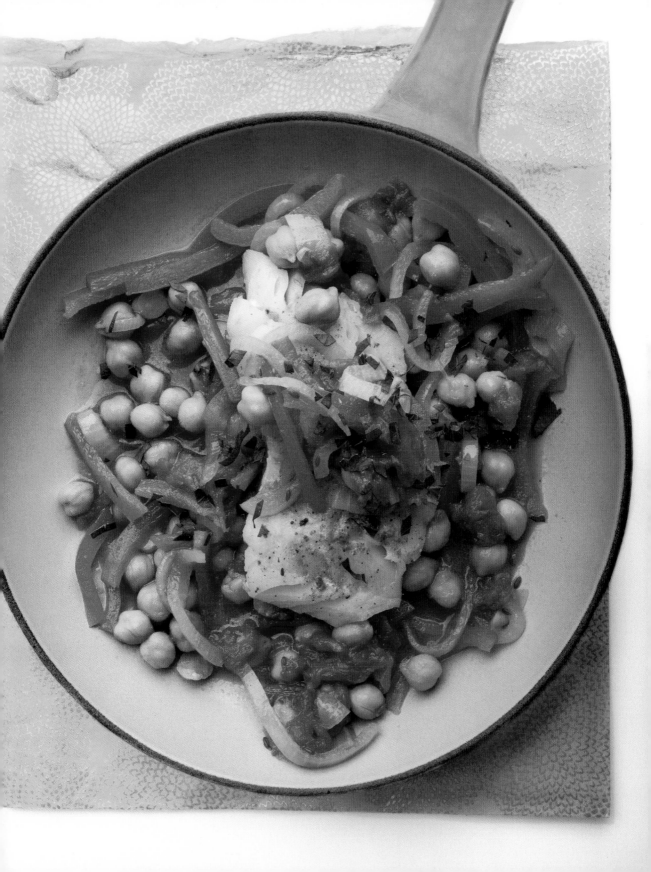

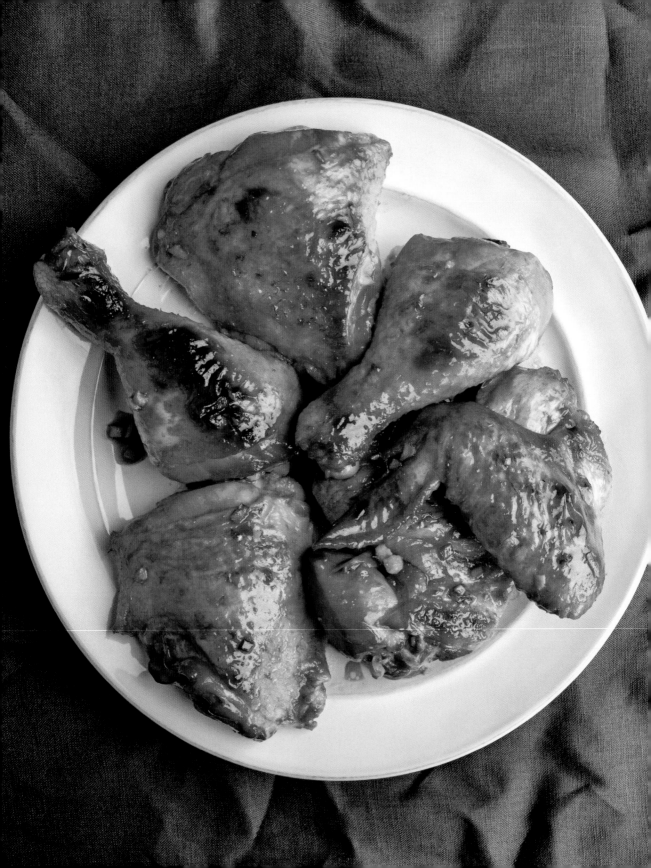

Soy-Glazed Chicken

HEALTH CONSIDERATIONS: IN TREATMENT; FATIGUE; LOW FIBER; GLUTEN-FREE; NEUTROPENIC DIET; HEALTHY SURVIVORSHIP; BLAND DIET

FOOD PREFERENCE: DAIRY-FREE

Meal: Main

Main Ingredient: Chicken

Prep Time: 15 minutes, plus 30 minutes for marinating

Cook Time: 30 minutes

SERVES 6

Teriyaki-style chicken is as easy to make as it is delicious. This zesty mix of salty and sweet spiked with grated ginger and lemon zest is guaranteed to eradicate the chemo blahs that can often make plain grilled chicken seem tasteless and even unpleasant. The longer the chicken can soak up the marinade, the better it will be, so plan ahead. Enjoy it with a crunchy salad or some quickly cooked greens (page 36).

Marinade

⅔ cup soy sauce (tamari for gluten-free)

1 tablespoon sugar

2 tablespoons extra-virgin olive oil

1 tablespoon peeled, chopped fresh gingerroot

2 cloves garlic, smashed and sliced

1 tablespoon cider vinegar

2 teaspoons grated lemon zest

1 free-range, organic chicken, skin on, cut into 8 pieces (see Ann's Tips, next page, if you're on a bland diet)

Scallions, thinly sliced and blanched, for garnish

1. Make the marinade: In a medium saucepan set over high heat, bring the soy sauce, sugar, oil, ginger, garlic, vinegar, and lemon zest to a boil. Once boiling, immediately remove from the heat.

2. Pat the chicken pieces dry and lay them in a dish just big enough to tightly hold them in one layer. Cover with the marinade, turning the pieces to ensure all are well coated. Cover with plastic wrap and leave in the refrigerator to marinate for as long as possible, but at least 1 hour. Turn the pieces every so often to make sure they are marinating evenly.

3. Preheat the oven to 400°F (see Ann's Tips, below). Line a baking sheet with foil for easy cleanup.

4. Place the chicken on the prepared baking sheet and set it under the broiler on a high rack. Brown the skin of the chicken pieces, basting with marinade and turning until they are lightly browned all over and no uncooked areas remain, 12 to 15 minutes total.

5. Transfer the baking sheet to a rack in the middle of the oven and bake, basting with the remaining marinade, for 10 to 14 minutes or until the juices run clear. When the chicken is ready, transfer to a warm dish, cover, and let rest for 5 to 10 minutes before serving. Serve sprinkled with blanched scallions.

Ann's Tips

· ✳ ·

If you are on a bland diet, ask your butcher to skin and cut the chicken for you.

Unless you're following a neutropenic diet, there's no need to blanch the scallions.

If your broiler is separate and has a more sophisticated heating system than your oven, preheat to medium-high and brown the chicken in step 4, and then move to the oven. However, if your broiler is like mine—at the bottom of my oven and pretty rudimentary, with only one temperature and two rack positions: high, which almost touches the flame, and low—I have found that I can regulate my broiler's temperature by using the higher range of the oven temperature. For this recipe, preheating the oven to 400°F will heat the broiler, too. This gentler, slower broiling temperature allows the chicken to brown in step 4 without charring. The chicken can then go straight into the oven to finish cooking in step 5.

Shepherd's Pie

HEALTH CONSIDERATIONS: IN TREATMENT; GLUTEN-FREE; NEUTROPENIC DIET; HEALTHY SURVIVORSHIP

FOOD PREFERENCE: NONE

Shepherd's pie was a staple of my British childhood. It is real comfort food for cold, damp English winter afternoons and long winter nights—American ones, too! In fact, I often make the filling to keep in my freezer for a quick cozy meal when I don't feel like cooking. To round out the influence of my years in the States, and for extra taste and nutrition, I've topped this pie with mashed sweet potatoes instead of Idaho potatoes. I don't miss the beef—turkey does the job just as well, and along with the more traditional peas, I've added some dark leafy greens. Any steamed dark greens—spinach, kale, or collards—made from scratch (page 36) will do, but since frozen are fast and convenient when you're tired, that's what we're using here. The Worcestershire sauce and Tabasco give the pie richness rather than heat, so don't hold back.

Meal: Lunch, Dinner

Main Ingredients: Turkey, Sweet potatoes

Prep Time: 30 minutes

Cook Time: 45 minutes

SERVES 4 TO 6

Topping

2 large red sweet potatoes, peeled and cut into 1-inch dice

½ teaspoon sea salt, or to taste

1 tablespoon butter, or to taste (see Ann's Tips, page 171)

Freshly grated nutmeg, to taste (optional)

Filling

2 tablespoons extra-virgin olive oil

1 pound ground turkey (see Ann's tips, page 171)

1 large yellow onion, diced

3 medium carrots, scrubbed and cut into small dice

2 stalks celery, cut into small dice

1 bay leaf

Sea salt and freshly ground black pepper, to taste

2 cloves garlic, smashed and chopped

(continued)

1 tablespoon tomato paste	2 whole sprigs flat-leaf parsley, plus 2 tablespoons chopped
1 cup water or Basic Vegetable Broth (page 21)	1 (10-ounce) package frozen chopped kale, collards, or leaf spinach
1 teaspoon Tabasco	½ cup frozen peas
1 tablespoon Worcestershire sauce, or to taste	Juice of ½ lemon

1. Grease an 11 x 7 x 2-inch (1½-quart) baking dish and set aside.

2. In a large pot, bring the diced sweet potatoes, salt, and enough water to cover to a boil. Once boiling, cover and lower the heat to medium. Cook for 20 minutes, or until the potatoes are tender enough to mash against the sides of the pan. Drain, return to the pot, and mash with the butter and a grind or two of nutmeg, if using. Taste for salt. Set aside on top of the stove to keep warm.

3. While the potatoes are cooking, heat the oil in a large sauté pan over medium-high heat. Add the ground turkey and cook for 5 minutes, or until there is no pink left and the meat has started to brown. Add the onion, carrots, celery, and bay leaf. Sprinkle with salt and cook for about 2 minutes, or until the onion starts to soften and turn translucent. Cover, reduce the heat to medium, and gently cook for 8 to 10 minutes, stirring occasionally to prevent the vegetables and meat from sticking.

4. Uncover the pan and increase the heat to medium-high. Add the garlic and a grind or two of black pepper. Sauté for 1 minute, or until you can smell the garlic's aroma. Add the tomato paste, stir to mix, and cook until it becomes orangey in color and begins to caramelize, about 2 minutes. Add the water and bring to a boil. Partially cover, reduce the heat to medium-low, and simmer for 10 minutes.

5. Add the Tabasco and Worcestershire sauce and stir to mix. Lay the 2 parsley sprigs on top and partially cover. Simmer for 10 to 15 minutes more or until the vegetables are just soft and the liquid has reduced by about half. Remove the parsley stems and discard.

6. Preheat the broiler with the rack in the low position.

7. Add the frozen greens, peas, and the chopped parsley to the turkey mixture. Cook, stirring to heat the veggies through for 3 to 5 minutes. Check for seasoning. Stir in the lemon juice. Spoon into the prepared baking dish. Cover with the reserved mashed sweet potato, making lines across the top with a fork. Drizzle with a little oil. Set under the broiler and cook until browned. Let it sit for 5 minutes on top of the stove. Serve.

Ann's Tips

· ✳ ·

To make the turkey filling for the freezer, make the recipe up to the end of step 4 and bag and freeze. All that's left to do for a 30-minute meal is to defrost the filling, make the mashed potato topping, and jump to step 5.

If you're cutting down on saturated fats, mash the potatoes with olive oil instead of butter. And for extra fiber, don't even peel the potatoes, just scrub, dice, and cook them, peel and all.

For an even faster topping, try a can of plain pumpkin puree beaten with a grating or two of nutmeg and 1 tablespoon olive oil.

If you are buying prepacked ground turkey, don't buy the "breast only" packs. They are less flavorful than the mixed. Most packs of commercially ground turkey are anywhere from 1 pound (16 ounces) to 1¼ pounds (20 ounces). If your pack is the larger size, use the whole thing.

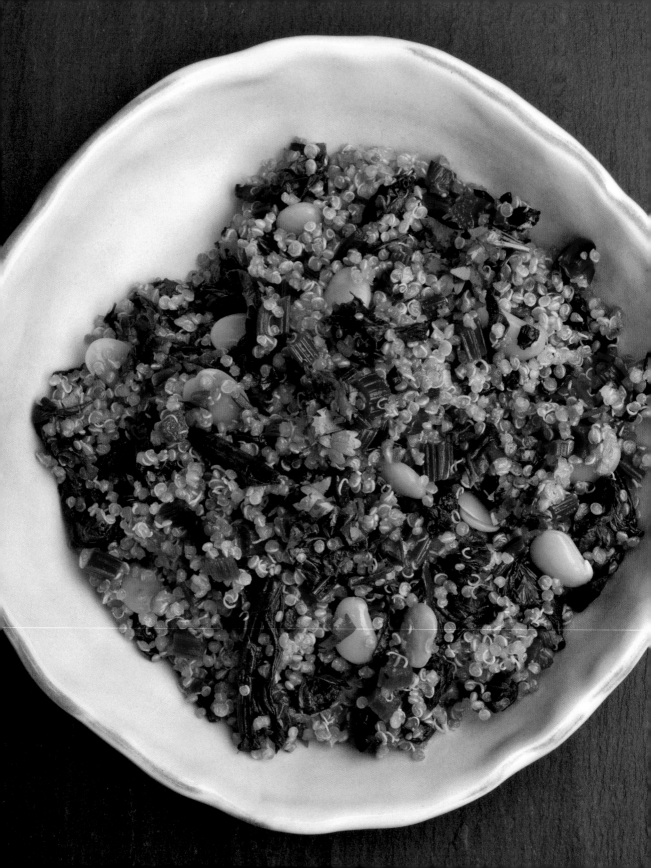

Spiced Quinoa with Beet Greens

HEALTH CONSIDERATIONS: IN TREATMENT; NAUSEA; GLUTEN-FREE; HIGH CALORIE; HEALTHY SURVIVORSHIP; NEUTROPENIC DIET

FOOD PREFERENCE: DAIRY-FREE; VEGAN; VEGETARIAN

Meal: Main, Side

Main Ingredient: Beets

Prep Time: 20 minutes

Cook Time: 15 to 20 minutes

SERVES 4

Beet greens are super vegetables. Bursting with vitamins A, C, and K plus a slew of minerals, they are among the most nutritious leafy vegetables you can eat. This quick one-pot meal is a great way to eat them. It combines protein-rich quinoa with every part of the greens—stems and leaves. And since the leaves are as tender as spinach, once you've stirred them in, the dish is pretty much done.

1 large bunch beets and their greens

2 tablespoons extra-virgin olive oil

1 dried red chili pepper, or to taste, seeds removed

½ teaspoon cumin seeds

1 teaspoon grated gingerroot

1 small red onion, finely diced (about ½ cup)

Sea salt, to taste

½ (14-ounce) can plum tomatoes, drained and chopped

2 cups cooked Basic Quinoa (page 33)

½ cup frozen baby lima beans

Juice of ½ lime

2 tablespoons chopped cilantro

1. Cut the greens from the beets. Reserve the beets for another use (Baltic Beet Salad, page 303, or Beet Risotto, page 299).
2. Wash the greens and strip the tender leaves from the stems. Slice the stems into a fine dice and roughly chop the greens. Set aside.
3. Heat the oil in a medium wok or sauté pan over medium-high heat. When the oil is hot, add the chili pepper, cumin, and ginger. Cook, stirring, until the cumin seeds darken, 30 seconds to 1 minute. Add the onion, diced beet stems, and a

sprinkle of salt. Stir and cook for 5 to 7 minutes, or until the vegetables start to soften.

4. Add the tomatoes and cook until they start to look saucy and turn slightly orange in color, about 3 minutes. Add the quinoa and mix well. Cook, stirring, until the quinoa is heated through and has started to absorb the cooking juices. Add the frozen lima beans and cook about 2 minutes, or until they start to soften. Taste for salt.

5. Add the chopped beet greens and stir until they wilt. Stir in the lime juice and cilantro and mix well. Cover and turn off the heat. Allow the mixture to sit for 2 minutes before serving.

Ann's Tips

· ☥ ·

Use ruby chard if you don't have beet greens, cutting the stems into a small dice.

Raw, unpeeled beets can last up to 2 weeks in the crisper drawer in your refrigerator.

Sautéed Spinach with Nutmeg

HEALTH CONSIDERATIONS: BLAND DIET; GLUTEN-FREE; IN TREATMENT; EASY TO SWALLOW; HEALTHY SURVIVORSHIP; FATIGUE; NEUTROPENIC DIET

FOOD PREFERENCE: VEGETARIAN

Meal: Side

Main Ingredient: Spinach

Prep Time: 10 minutes

Cook Time: 5 to 8 minutes

SERVES 2

This was how my mom used to cook spinach. Every time I eat spinach this way, I think of her! She would have loved to have had baby spinach to use instead of the sturdier, large leaf spinach we had in the UK. The washing and prep for that takes three times longer than the cooking. With baby spinach, there's far less muss and fuss, but to be on the safe side, particularly if you're on chemo, wash the leaves in a salad spinner before cooking even if the package declares it prewashed. And cook the spinach in butter—don't substitute, since it's the butter that makes this simple dish so very delicious.

2 (5-ounce bags) baby spinach

1 tablespoon unsalted butter

1 clove garlic, peeled and smashed

½ teaspoon freshly grated nutmeg, or to taste (see Ann's Tips, next page)

Sea salt, to taste

1. In a wide saucepan or sauté pan, heat the butter over medium-high heat until it foams. Add the garlic, reduce the heat to medium, and cook, stirring, until the garlic starts to turn golden, about 3 minutes. Don't let either the garlic or the butter burn.
2. Add the grated nutmeg and let it sizzle for 30 seconds, then turn the heat back up to medium-high and add the spinach, a few handfuls at a time, along with a sprinkle of sea salt. The pan will get full quickly, so stir the spinach as you go, adding more as it wilts, which it will do almost immediately. Once all the spinach is in and is completely wilted, discard the garlic and taste for salt. Serve immediately.

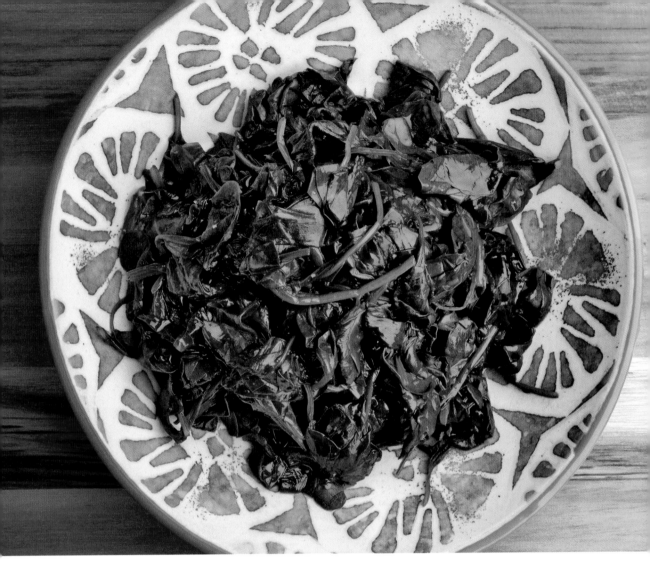

Allow 5 ounces of baby spinach per person. Like celery, baby spinach is on the "Dirty Dozen" list, so buy organic if you can.

I happen to love nutmeg, but if you are unfamiliar with using it, start with half the amount suggested here. You can always add more.

Vegetable Salad à la Niçoise

HEALTH CONSIDERATIONS: IN TREATMENT; GLUTEN-FREE; HIGH FIBER; HEALTHY SURVIVORSHIP; NEUTROPENIC DIET

FOOD PREFERENCE: DAIRY-FREE; VEGETARIAN

Meal: Side, Salad

Main Ingredients: Beans, Potatoes, Olives

Prep Time: 30 minutes

Cook Time: 20 minutes

SERVES 4 TO 6

This is a real *salade composée*. It has many parts, all cooked, and is a meal in itself. Besides being a summery delicious meal, the other good thing about it is that it is a tasty, safe salad for an antimicrobial diet. With all the different things to cook, it can seem a little fiddly, but the potatoes can steam while tomatoes roast and all can be thrown together in the dressing at the last minute.

1½ cups cherry tomatoes (see Ann's Tips, next page)

2 teaspoons extra-virgin olive oil

6 to 8 small round Yukon Gold or Red Bliss potatoes, scrubbed

½ pound French beans or green beans, washed, trimmed, and cut into 1-inch pieces

2 small carrots, scrubbed and cut into a thick julienne about the width and length of the beans

2 or 3 large Soft- or Hard-Boiled Eggs (page 29), peeled and quartered

½ cup small oil-cured black olives

8 to 10 basil leaves gently torn (optional; see Ann's Tips, next page)

Sea salt, to taste

Mustard Vinaigrette

1 tablespoon Dijon mustard

Sea salt and freshly ground black pepper, to taste

1 tablespoon white wine vinegar

3 tablespoons extra-virgin olive oil

1 tablespoon water

1. Preheat the oven to 425°F. Line a baking sheet with parchment paper and place on a rack in the upper third of the oven.
2. Put the tomatoes and oil together in a bowl. Toss to coat. Tip onto the preheated baking sheet and bake for 15 to 20 minutes. Set aside.

3. Meanwhile, put the potatoes into a saucepan with just enough water to cover and a pinch of salt. Bring to a boil over high heat. Reduce the heat to medium and cook until the potatoes are tender, 15 to 20 minutes, depending on their size. A knife point should slip into the largest potato smoothly. Steam the beans and carrots for 5 minutes. To save a pan and time, I usually do this over the potatoes toward the end of their cooking time. Drain all the vegetables and shock them in cold water to stop them from cooking more. When you can handle them, halve or quarter the potatoes, depending on their size, discarding any skin that slips off. Set aside.

4. Make the vinaigrette in a large salad bowl: Beat the mustard and vinegar together until smooth. Add a pinch of salt and a grind or two of black pepper. Gradually add the oil, beating constantly until you have a creamy sauce. Taste for salt and acidity. Beat in the water, 1 teaspoon at a time, if the dressing is too thick.

5. Add the potatoes, beans, roasted cherry tomatoes, and the olives to the dressing and toss together until well mixed and covered in the dressing. Allow to sit for 10 minutes so the flavors can develop. Serve topped with boiled-egg pieces and scattered torn basil leaves.

Ann's Tips

· ⌖ ·

If you are on a neutropenic diet, you will need to cook the basil leaves. To make the most of their flavor, in a small skillet or saucepan, heat 1 to 2 tablespoons of the oil set aside for the dressing over a medium-low heat. When hot, add the torn basil leaves and cook for 3 minutes. This will flavor the oil and deal with any microbes. Use this flavored oil, basil leaves included, to make the salad dressing. And if this is too much work, simply add half a teaspoon of commercial jarred pesto to the dressing.

Although they taste great, you don't need to roast the tomatoes if you can eat raw foods. Skip step 2 and just halve the tomatoes to toss with the cooked vegetables.

If/when you can eat them, you can serve the salad heaped on a bed of crisp romaine lettuce or other salad greens.

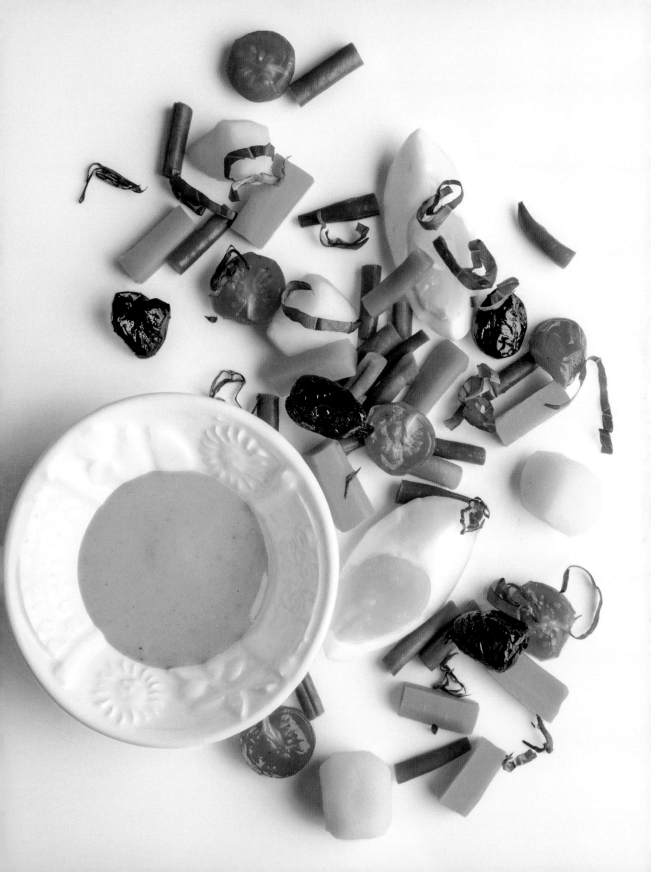

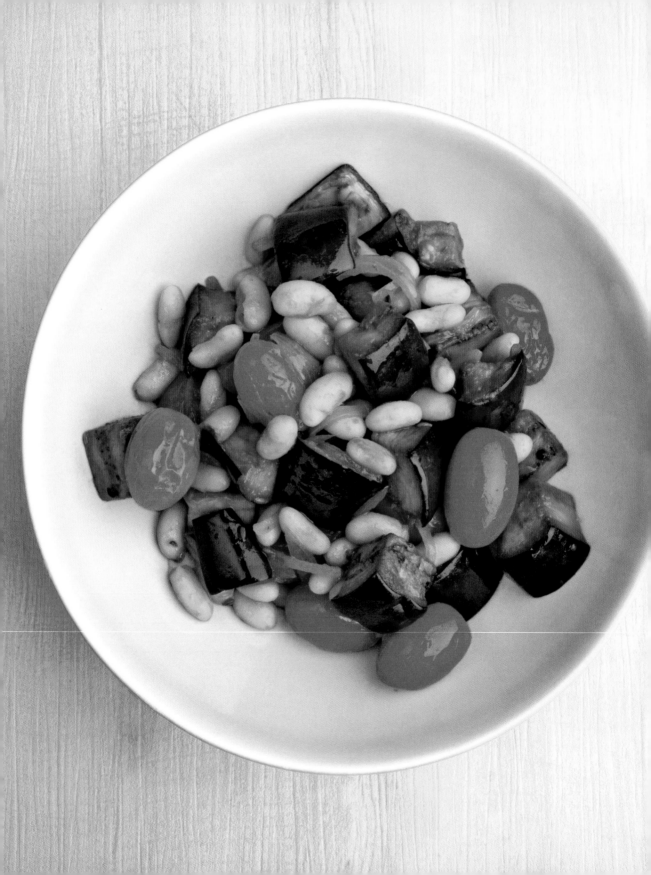

Roasted Eggplant and White Bean Stew

Meal: Side

Main Ingredient:
Eggplant, Tomatoes

Prep Time: 20 minutes

Cook Time: 40 minutes

SERVES 2 TO 4

HEALTH CONSIDERATIONS: IN TREATMENT; FATIGUE; HIGH FIBER; GLUTEN-FREE; NEUTROPENIC DIET; HEALTHY SURVIVORSHIP

FOOD PREFERENCE: DAIRY-FREE; VEGAN; VEGETARIAN

This is an easy, late-summer dish and totally delicious either hot or cold. Its deep roasted flavors lifted by a squeeze of lemon juice are a great foil to the vagaries of taste bud changes during treatment. It is a nutrient-dense dish, too. Although it seems to have a lot of moving parts, there's not a huge amount of actual prep. If you work while the eggplant and tomatoes are roasting, things will come together very quickly.

2 tablespoons extra-virgin olive oil, divided

2 small Italian eggplants, halved and cut into 1-inch chunks (see Ann's Tips, page 183)

1 teaspoon sea salt, or to taste

2 cups grape tomatoes

1 teaspoon cumin seeds

1 clove garlic, thinly sliced

1 bay leaf

1 hot dried red pepper, deseeded and broken into pieces (optional and to taste)

1 (1-inch) piece gingerroot, peeled, julienned, and then diced

2 shallots, halved and thinly sliced through the root end

1 teaspoon tomato paste

½ cup water or Basic Vegetable Broth (page 21)

1 (14-ounce) can cannellini beans, drained and rinsed (see Ann's Tips, page 183)

Lemon wedges, to garnish

1. Preheat the oven to 425°F. Line a baking sheet with parchment paper and let it heat in the oven for 10 minutes before using.

2. Pour 2 teaspoons of the oil into a large bowl. Add the eggplant, sprinkle with ½ teaspoon of the salt, and mix until all the pieces are coated in oil. Tip the eggplant onto the prepared baking sheet in a single layer, cut-sides down, leaving room for the tomatoes at one end. Add another 1 teaspoon of the oil to the bowl and add the tomatoes. Turn gently to coat and tip onto the baking sheet in one layer. Drizzle any oil remaining in the bowl over the eggplant. Roast the vegetables on a rack set in the upper third of the oven for 20 to 25 minutes, turning them after 15 minutes. They will be slightly browned and caramelized. Set aside.

3. While the vegetables are roasting, heat the remaining oil in a wide, shallow saucepan. Add the cumin and let it sizzle for 30 seconds, then add the garlic, bay leaf, hot pepper, if using, and the ginger. Cook, stirring, until the garlic starts to color, 2 to 3 minutes. Add the shallots. Sprinkle with salt and lower the heat to medium. Cook until the shallots start to caramelize, 5 to 8 minutes.

4. Mix the tomato paste into the shallots. Cook until it starts to turn a deep orangey-red, about 1 minute. Add the water and bring to a simmer. Add the beans. Stir to mix, cover, and cook until the beans are heated through and tender, about 5 minutes. Add the roasted eggplant, stir to mix, then add the tomatoes. Gently stir to mix. Cover and cook over low heat for 15 minutes for the flavors to blend. Turn the heat off and let the stew sit for 10 minutes. Taste for salt. Serve warm or at room temperature with lemon wedges.

Larger, older eggplants sometimes have bitter juices, so they are often salted. Salt makes the cut slices bead with "sweat," which draws this bitterness out. I usually look to buy either skinny Asian eggplants that never need salting or the smaller-size Italian eggplants that are hard and firm to the touch, so that salting isn't necessary. But if you aren't sure about the age of your eggplant, cube it as per the recipe, transfer to a colander, and toss with salt. Leave to drain in the sink for 30 minutes. Rinse off the salt and pat the eggplant dry before tossing in oil and roasting.

If you make your own white beans from scratch (page 40), use them here instead of canned. Drain them, reserving a half cup of their cooking liquid to use instead of the water.

Ann's Tips

· ✳ ·

Summer Sauté

Meal: Side

Main Ingredients:
Tomatoes, Zucchini, Corn

Prep Time: 30 minutes

Cook Time: 20 minutes

SERVES 2 TO 4

HEALTH CONSIDERATIONS: IN TREATMENT; FATIGUE; HIGH FIBER; GLUTEN-FREE; NEUTROPENIC DIET; HEALTHY SURVIVORSHIP

FOOD PREFERENCE: DAIRY-FREE; VEGAN; VEGETARIAN

The taste of this dish lies in the cooking. Don't crowd the pan. You want the green vegetables to sauté, not steam, so give them the room and the time to lightly brown and caramelize before you add the tomatoes. The sweetness that comes out of them is the key to this simple dish.

1 tablespoon extra-virgin olive oil

3 scallions, diced

1 stalk celery, finely diced

2 small zucchini or summer squash, deseeded and finely diced

Sea salt, to taste

1 ear corn, shucked and kernels stripped (see Ann's Tips, next page)

1 medium ripe beefsteak tomato or 2 ripe Roma tomatoes, diced (see Ann's Tips, next page)

¼ cup torn basil leaves

1 to 2 teaspoons lemon juice

1. Heat the oil in a medium sauté pan over medium-high heat. Once it's hot, add the scallions, celery, zucchini, and a sprinkle of sea salt. Cook, stirring occasionally, for 10 minutes, or until vegetables start to soften and caramelize.

2. Add the corn kernels and cook for 2 minutes, stirring all the while. Add the tomatoes and cook, stirring often, for 5 to 8 minutes, or until the tomatoes start to look saucy.

3. Add the basil leaves and lemon juice and mix to combine. Serve immediately.

Use grape tomatoes early in the season, when they have more flavor.

Use 1 cup frozen corn kernels when corn is out of season.

If you are on a neutropenic diet, add the basil and cook for 2 minutes before adding the lemon juice and eating.

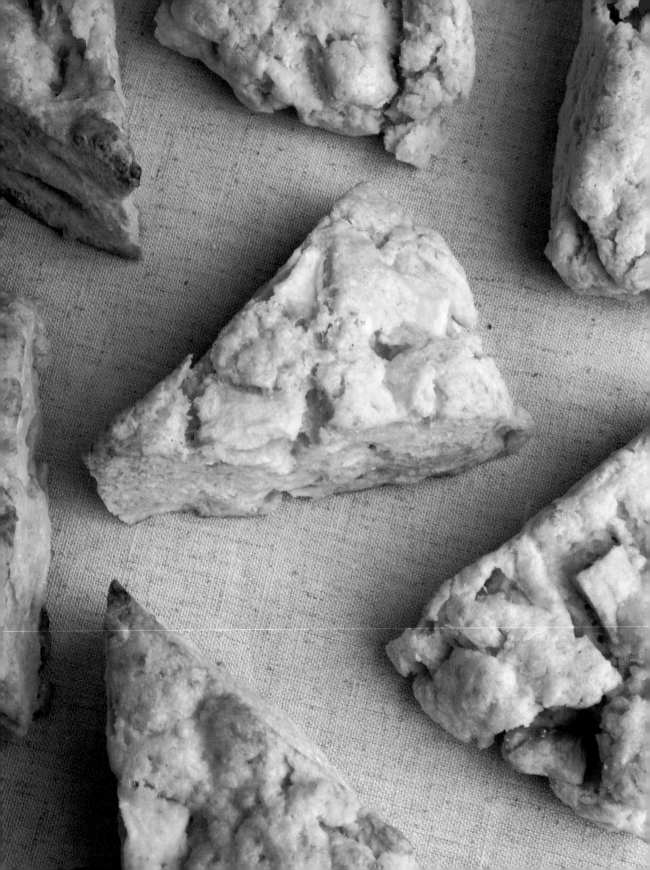

Apple-Cheddar Scones

HEALTH CONSIDERATIONS: IN TREATMENT; FATIGUE; BLAND DIET; NEUTROPENIC DIET, NAUSEA

FOOD PREFERENCE: VEGETARIAN

Scones are so easy to throw together that I'm always amazed when people buy them. They freeze well, too, so you don't need a cast of thousands to eat a batch. These cheesy, savory treats get a hint of sweetness from the chunks of apple. They are a fabulous quick snack when you're lacking the energy to eat much and don't want to dive into the cookie jar. You can eat them as is, or split and toast them. Yummy either way.

Meal: Snack

Main Ingredients: Whole-wheat flour, Cheese, Apples

Prep Time: 20 minutes

Cook Time: 10 to 15 minutes

MAKES 8 SCONES

1 cup whole-wheat pastry flour

1 cup unbleached all-purpose white flour

2 teaspoons baking powder

½ teaspoon sea salt

½ teaspoon freshly grated nutmeg

1 tablespoon fine brown sugar

3 tablespoons cold unsalted butter, diced

1 cup grated cheddar

1 large egg

Milk, as needed

2 small apples or 1 large, peeled, cored, and cut into ¼-inch dice

1. Preheat the oven to 400°F.
2. Sift together the flours, baking powder, salt, and nutmeg in a large bowl. Stir in the sugar. Rub in the butter with the tips of your fingers, or pulse the mixture together in a food processor, until it resembles coarse bread crumbs. Stir in the grated cheddar.
3. Break the egg into a 2-cup measuring jug. Add enough milk to bring the egg mixture to ½ cup. Beat together lightly.
4. Make a well in the dry ingredients and add the egg mixture. Mix together with a spatula or a fork until it forms a soft dough. Fold in the diced apple and knead

lightly to form a ball. If the dough seems dry, add more milk, 1 tablespoon at a time.

5. Roll out the dough on a floured surface into a disk a little more than 1 inch thick. Place the disk on a lightly floured cookie sheet. Cut it into 8 wedges and gently push the wedges apart to separate them. The wedges will need room to spread and rise. Bake for 10 to 15 minutes in the upper third of the oven. Cool slightly on a wire rack and eat warm. Freeze or store in an airtight container.

Ann's Tips

·✳·

These scones also make for a pretty good cheesy treat without the apples.

If you want to make a lower-fiber scone, cut the whole-wheat flour and use unbleached all-purpose flour.

If you have whole-wheat pastry flour on hand, instead of mixing the flours, use 2 cups of whole-wheat pastry flour.

Stewed Prunes

HEALTH CONSIDERATIONS: IN TREATMENT; EASY TO SWALLOW; NAUSEA; HIGH FIBER; GLUTEN-FREE; NEUTROPENIC DIET; HEALTHY SURVIVORSHIP

FOOD PREFERENCE: DAIRY-FREE; VEGAN; VEGETARIAN

Meal: Dessert

Main Ingredient: Prunes

Prep Time: 5 minutes

Cook Time: 30 minutes

SERVES 4 TO 6

I used to hate prunes. Really hate them. They reminded me of bad school lunches. That was until I started to travel in Italy for work. In the restaurants, the dessert trolleys would trundle by after lunch laden with tarts, cakes, gelato, and, surprisingly, large bowls of prunes. These didn't look like school lunches, so eventually I tried them. Unexpected deliciousness in a light, lemony syrup! Hate turned to love! Here they are for you, with all the "good for you" fiber and vitamins that come with them.

1 to 1½ pounds large whole prunes (see Ann's Tips, next page)

1 small lemon, halved

3 tablespoons maple syrup or organic granulated cane sugar, to taste

1. Place the prunes and lemon halves in a nonreactive pot over medium-high heat. Drizzle with the maple syrup and add enough water to just cover the fruit. Bring to a boil.
2. Cover and turn the heat down to low, then simmer gently for 30 to 35 minutes, turning the prunes every so often and adding water if they look too dry. The liquid will be syrupy and the prunes will have softened and swelled up when ready.
3. Remove from the heat and let the prunes cool. Transfer to a container. They will keep refrigerated for up to 1 week, if they last that long! Eat them as is or with a dollop of Greek yogurt.

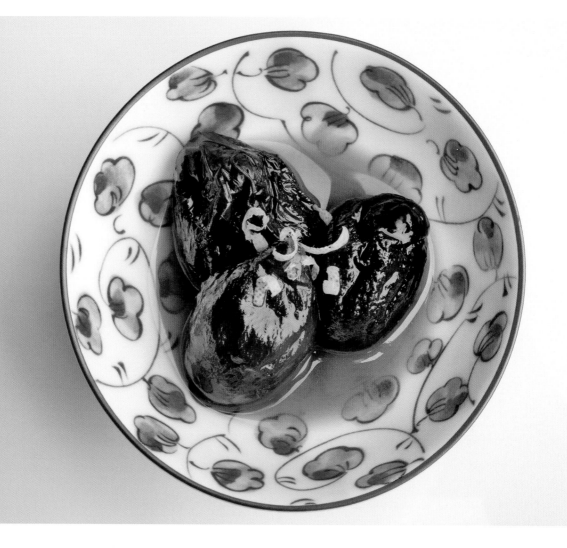

Buy whole prunes, not pitted. Prunes should be soft, sticky, and a little glossy look-ing. If yours are tough and look dried out, soak them in hot water for 1 hour to plump them before cooking. My favorites are the delicious French prunes that come from Agen in Southwest France. Look for them in your specialty market. Avoid jumbo prunes, however; these are often dried round black plums and have a completely different flavor.

Jamaican Sorrel Tea

Meal: Beverages

Main Ingredients: Hibiscus flowers, Ginger

Prep Time: 5 minutes

Cook Time: 5-plus minutes to steep (see Ann's Tips, below)

MAKES 1½ QUARTS

HEALTH CONSIDERATIONS: IN TREATMENT; FATIGUE; NAUSEA; BLAND DIET; LOW FIBER: GLUTEN-FREE; EASY TO SWALLOW; HEALTHY SURVIVORSHIP; NEUTROPENIC DIET

FOOD PREFERENCE: DAIRY-FREE; VEGAN; VEGETARIAN

This is a great drink to have during chemo treatment. Sorrel is the Jamaican name for the hibiscus flowers that are in season around Christmastime. This traditional drink combines the tastes of hibiscus and ginger, a partnership truly made in heaven. Dried hibiscus flowers have a wonderful, tart taste that pleasantly neutralizes any bad taste from chemo drugs, while ginger brings spiciness as it cools the body and aids in digestion. This glorious, naturally ruby-red tea is rich in vitamin C, beta-carotene, and antioxidant flavonoids.

¼ cup dried hibiscus flowers

1 (2-inch) piece gingerroot, thinly sliced (about 20 slices)

1 (1-inch) strip lemon zest

2 whole allspice

2 tablespoons agave nectar or honey, or to taste

6 to 8 cups boiling water

1. Put the dried hibiscus flowers, ginger, lemon zest, and allspice into a large pot. Cover with the boiling water and steep for 5 minutes or to desired strength.
2. Strain the tea into a jug or carafe through a fine sieve. It will be a gorgeous dark red. Stir in the agave or honey, to taste. Serve hot or over ice.

Ann's Tips

You can find dried hibiscus flowers at most health food stores, and at many specialty markets, particularly Latino markets, where they are known, unsurprisingly, as *flor de Jamaica* or Jamaican flowers.

For a stronger drink, leave the tea to steep overnight in the fridge before straining.

Spicy

· · · · ✈ · · · ·

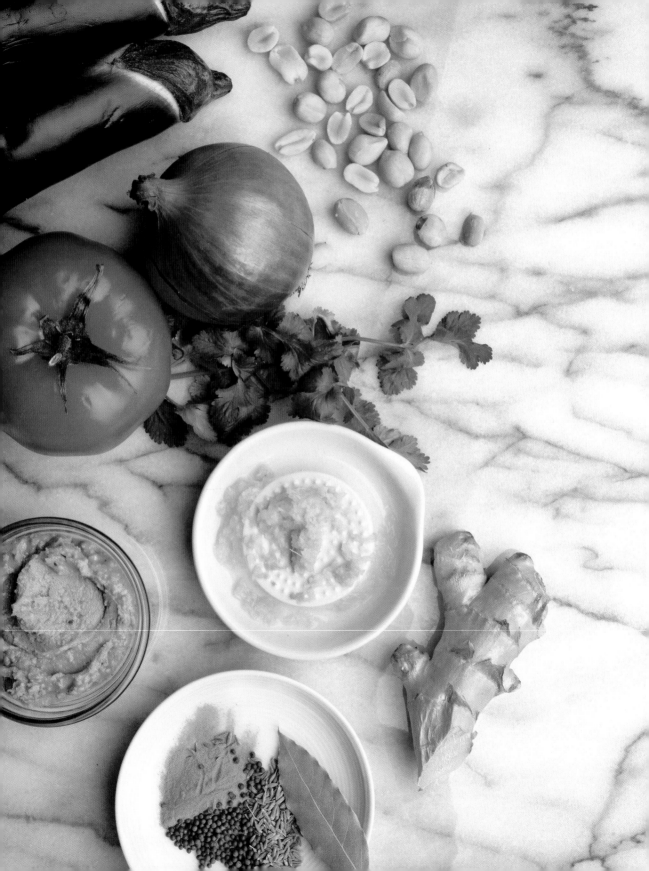

Taste change, or "chemo palate," is the most significant treatment side effect that you may not have heard of. Most people understand that they will lose their hair or get nausea when they go on chemo, but the loss of your sense of taste is something a lot of patients are not ready for—and some lose their sense of smell, too. Taste buds are fast-growing cells, and the chemo zaps them as surely as it zaps your hair follicles. You start to have difficulty distinguishing different tastes, and the results can be surprising, and often unpleasant. Overnight, your favorite foods become inedible; coffee undrinkable; sugar bitter; and clean, crisp water about as refreshing as mineral oil. What to do? Unfortunately this is the cancer patient's dilemma.

It's important to eat well during treatment to keep your weight up, but when your sense of taste goes, it's not so easy. When my taste buds started to play tricks on me, I decided it was time to experiment in the kitchen to see what worked best to fight against this unpleasant side effect. It wasn't what I'd expected. For me, the answer lay in eating the hottest, strongest-tasting, spiciest foods possible. And I wasn't alone. I discovered that several of my chemo friends felt the same way. We found that strong, spicy flavors successfully counteracted the worst effects of chemo palate. From then on, if it was hot and spicy, we ate it. As our fatigue and nausea faded in between infusions, we sought out all international temples of spiciness that are Indian, Thai, Korean, and Mexican restaurants. We loved it. And it kept us strong.

Among the following recipes, although there are a lot of spicy, easy curries, I also use spices for flavor only, without adding any heat. If hot, spicy food isn't for you, just using sweet spices can make a huge difference in how food tastes to a chemo-impaired palate, plus it's good to get to know how to use them. Many spices, gentle turmeric being the best known, have cancer-protective properties and are worth getting to know beyond the exciting taste experiences they can give. With deliciously spicy meal ideas, both hot and sweet, along with some cool, re-freshing beverages to wash them down with, we will help you light a spark in the most jaded chemo palate, and maybe start a flavor love affair that will last long past your last treatment.

DON'T CHASE THE TASTE

At CFYL cooking classes, I often tell our students to avoid "chasing" the taste of favor-ite foods that no longer taste good as you can end up with a taste memory that could ruin your enjoyment of them for all time. In my experience it's better to wait until your chemo is over before tucking into your favorites again, as they won't taste right until chemo's over and done with. In the meantime, since comparisons are odious, even in the kitchen, it's best to try something new.

SOME LIKE IT HOT

Spiciness as in heat is a personal preference. In all our recipes you can adjust the heat to suit your needs. If you like it milder, use less cayenne; if you're using fresh chilies, make sure you cut out all the seeds and white pith, and if they're dried, crack them and shake out all the seeds.

HOW TO USE

Some basic ways to use spices: Whole spices can be added to the oil at the begin-ning of the cooking and toasted to give the oil flavor before adding the vegetables. Ground spices are delicate and burn easily. Add them to the vegetables at the end of their sautéing period and cook them for a minute before adding any liquid.

Smoky Black Bean Chili with Farro

Meal: Main

Main Ingredients: Black beans, Farro

Prep Time: 15 minutes

Cook Time: 50 minutes

SERVES 4

HEALTH CONSIDERATIONS: IN TREATMENT; HIGH FIBER; HEALTHY SURVIVORSHIP; NEUTROPENIC DIET

FOOD PREFERENCE: DAIRY-FREE; VEGAN; VEGETARIAN

This vegan chili will suit meat eaters and vegans alike. The farro not only gives the chili a chewy, meaty quality, but, with the beans, it also offers complete protein, making this a really satisfying one-pot meal. And if that's not enough, it's super easy to make, too.

Health Tip

If you are on a neutropenic diet, you will need to add the cilantro and jalapeño garnishes to the chili and cook for 3 minutes. And check with your doctor about how she feels about your eating probiotic yogurt during treatment.

1 cup farro

2 tablespoons extra-virgin olive oil

1 teaspoon cumin seeds (see Ann's Tips, next page)

3 cloves garlic, sliced

1 or 2 dried red chilies, or ½ teaspoon chili flakes (optional)

1 large Spanish onion, diced

1 poblano pepper, diced

1 bay leaf

½ teaspoon dried oregano

Sea salt, to taste

1 tablespoon tomato paste

1 (28-ounce) can diced tomatoes

1 dried chipotle pepper, or to taste

2 to 3 cups Basic Vegetable Broth (page 21) or water

3 sprigs cilantro

2 (14-ounce) cans black beans, drained and rinsed

Generous squeeze of lime juice

Garnishes: Chopped cilantro and jalapeño; quarters of a lime; Greek yogurt (see Ann's Tips, next page)

1. Rinse the farro, tip into a bowl, and cover with 2 cups of water. Leave to soak while you prepare and cook the vegetables through step 2.

2. Heat the oil in a large Dutch oven over medium-high heat. Add the cumin, let it sizzle, then add the garlic and red chili, if using. Sauté until the garlic starts to color, about 1 minute. Add the onion, poblano, bay leaf, and oregano. Sprinkle with sea salt and gently cook until the onion and pepper are soft and starting to caramelize.

3. Drain the farro and add to the vegetables. Cook, stirring, until it is coated in oil and well mixed into the vegetables. Stir in the tomato paste and cook until it starts to caramelize. Add the tomatoes and dried chipotle pepper. Cook until the tomatoes start to turn orangey-red, about 5 minutes. Add the stock, bring to a boil, then drape the cilantro stems on top, cover, and simmer for 20 minutes or until the farro is just becoming tender.

4. Push the cilantro to one side and mix in the beans. Simmer, covered, for 20 minutes, adding a little water if the chili looks too dry. The farro will have a soft and chewy texture. Discard the cilantro stems, stir in the lime juice, and allow the chili to sit for 5 minutes. Serve with the suggested garnishes (see Ann's Tips, below).

Ann's
Tips

You can soak the farro overnight if you desire; this will cut the cooking time down by about 10 minutes.

If you have only ground cumin, add it at the end of step 2. Sprinkle the cumin powder over the softened vegetables and stir to mix. Continue with step 3.

If your throat is sore, you may want to pass on the lime juice. Its acidity can irritate. To get the taste, zest half a lime, stir it into the chili in step 4, and cook 2 minutes.

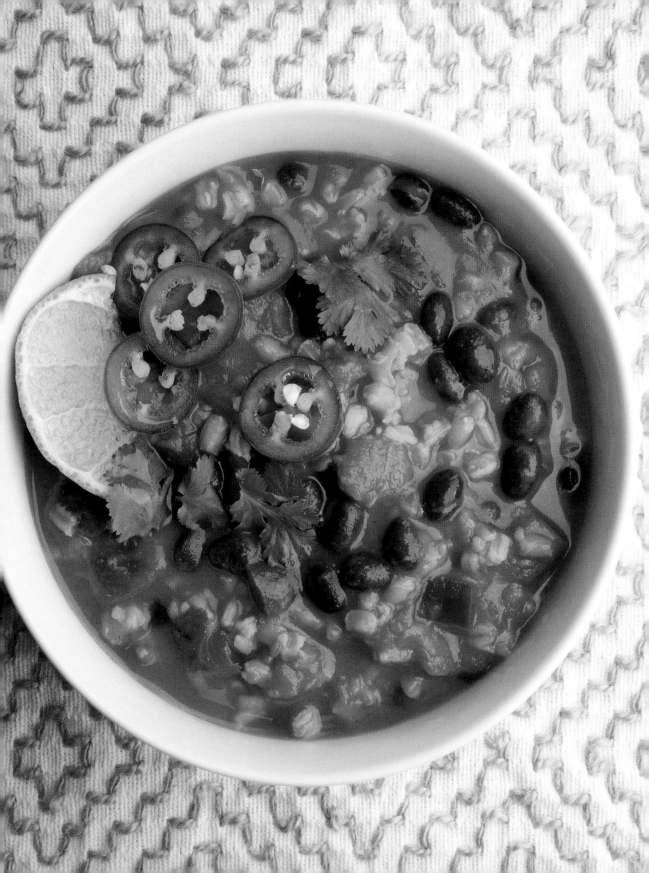

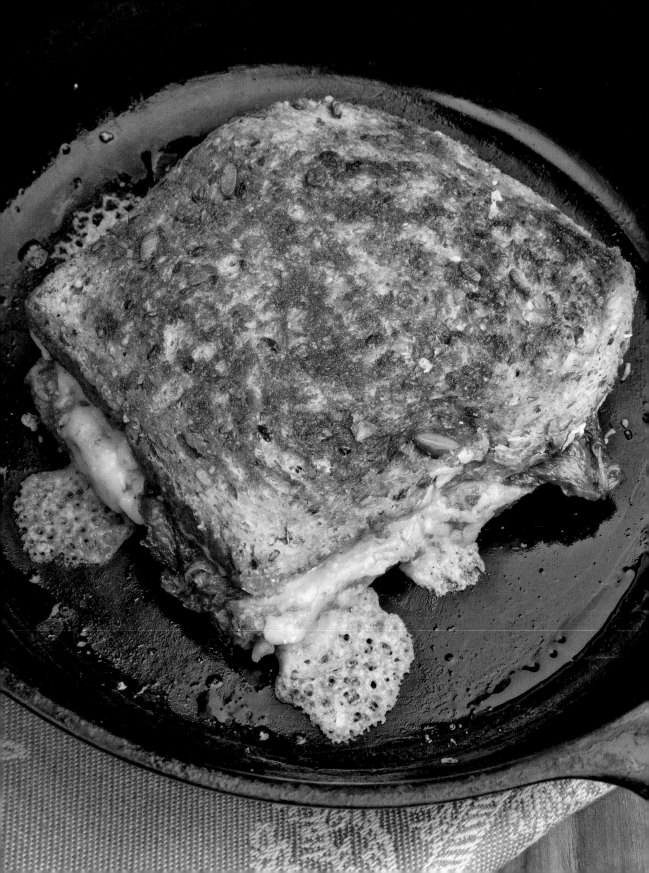

Kimchi Grilled Cheese Sandwich

HEALTH CONSIDERATIONS: IN TREATMENT; FATIGUE

FOOD PREFERENCE: VEGETARIAN

Meal: Main

Main Ingredients:
Cheese, Kimchi,
Whole-grain bread

Prep Time: 10 minutes

Cook Time: 10 minutes

SERVES 1

Kimchi is a spicy Korean pickle made with cabbage and other vegetables. Along with cancer-fighting cabbage, it is chock-full of antioxidant-rich garlic and chili peppers, and, most important, it's a great probiotic and it aids digestion. Kimchi may seem like an unusual ingredient to incorporate into everyday meals, but this sandwich is a great way to learn to love it. This tasty, nutritious twist on a classic comfort food isn't exactly the healthiest thing in the book, but sometimes a grilled cheese hits the mark. I call it healthy for the soul. I encourage you to give this delicious sandwich a try, and get some kimchi into your life!

Unsalted butter at room temperature or extra-virgin olive oil, to taste

2 slices whole-grain sourdough or other whole-grain bread of your choice

2 ounces good melting cheese like Gruyère, Emmenthal, or aged cheddar, thinly sliced or grated

1 tablespoon cabbage kimchi, or to taste

1. Heat a heavy-bottomed skillet over medium heat.
2. Butter, or brush with oil, one side of each bread slice.
3. Lay half the cheese on the dry side of one slice. Spread on the kimchi and layer the remaining cheese on top. Lay the remaining slice of bread on top, butter-side up, and press together.
4. Lay the sandwich in the heated skillet. When it is golden on the bottom, flip it and toast the other side, pressing the sandwich together as it cooks and the

cheese melts (see Ann's Tips, below). When it is golden, toasty, and the cheese is melted, eat immediately.

Ann's Tips

· ✙ ·

Kimchi is most commonly made from cabbage. It can be found in Asian markets, but thanks to its current popularity, stores like Trader Joe's and Whole Foods now carry it. You can often find it at farmers' markets, too, made from all kinds of vegetables. Also see Resources on page 328.

If you don't have kimchi on hand, or can't find it, use drained sauerkraut and a smidge of sriracha sauce instead.

If you have problems digesting milk products, you may be able to tolerate this with Pecorino Romano. It's made from sheep's milk and contains less lactose. Plus, it melts well.

Depending on the cheese, you may need to use the pan lid to circulate heat to help it melt.

Mushroom and Poblano Pepper Frittata

Meal: Main

Main Ingredient: Eggs, Mushrooms, Poblano peppers

Prep Time: 30 minutes

Cook Time: 25 minutes

SERVES 6 TO 8

HEALTH CONSIDERATIONS: IN TREATMENT; FATIGUE; GLUTEN-FREE; NEUTROPENIC DIET; HEALTHY SURVIVORSHIP

FOOD PREFERENCE: VEGETARIAN

Frittatas are wonderful standbys. Not only are they delicious eaten hot or cold, but also you can squeeze a lot of different ingredients into them. This one is a powerhouse of great cancer-fighting ingredients: mineral- and vitamin D–rich mushrooms, spicy poblanos with vitamin C, calcium from the cheese, antibacterial cilantro, etcetera, etcetera. And let's not forget the pumpkin seeds, either. I like best, though, that they are 1) easy to make and 2) taste amazing. The rest is icing.

2 tablespoons extra-virgin olive oil, divided

1 small red onion, sliced

2 large cloves garlic, peeled, smashed, and chopped

Sea salt, to taste

8 ounces mixed mushrooms, sliced

1 large poblano pepper, deseeded and diced

6 large eggs

2 tablespoons chopped fresh cilantro

½ teaspoon ground cumin

½ cup crumbled goat cheese, divided

½ cup pumpkin seeds

1. Preheat the oven to 400°F.
2. In an ovenproof, 10-inch skillet, heat 1 tablespoon of the oil over medium heat. Add the onion, garlic, and a pinch of salt and cook, stirring, for 6 minutes, or until softened and brown. Transfer to a plate and set aside.
3. In the same skillet, heat the remaining 1 tablespoon of oil over medium-high heat. Add the mushrooms and poblano. Cook, stirring, for about 5 minutes, or

until the mushrooms have wilted and are beginning to brown. Remove the skillet from the heat.

4. In a medium bowl, whisk the eggs with cilantro, cumin, and a pinch of salt.

5. Return the onion mixture back to the skillet over the mushrooms. Top with half the cheese. Pour the egg mixture over the vegetables and top with the remaining cheese and the pumpkin seeds.

6. Bake in the oven for 8 to 10 minutes or until the eggs are set and the cheese is slightly browned. If the top isn't completely cooked you can finish the frittata off under the broiler until just a pale gold, about 3 minutes. Keep watch—you don't want it to burn. To serve, run a heatproof spatula around the edge of the skillet and cut into wedges.

Ann's Tips

· 🐦 ·

If you can't find poblano peppers, use an Italian frying pepper or a sweet green pepper. With both, add 1 diced jalapeño to give spice and flavor.

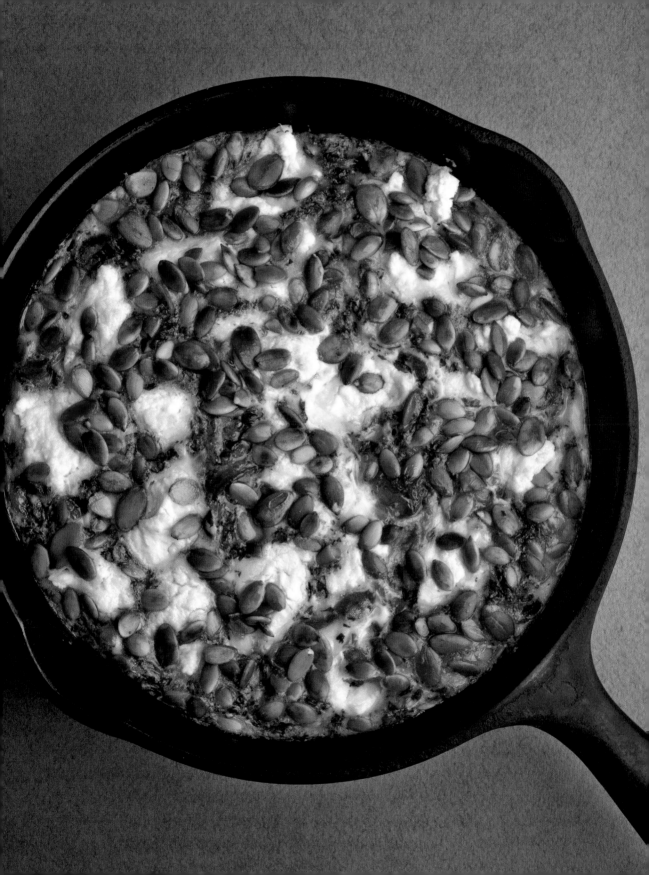

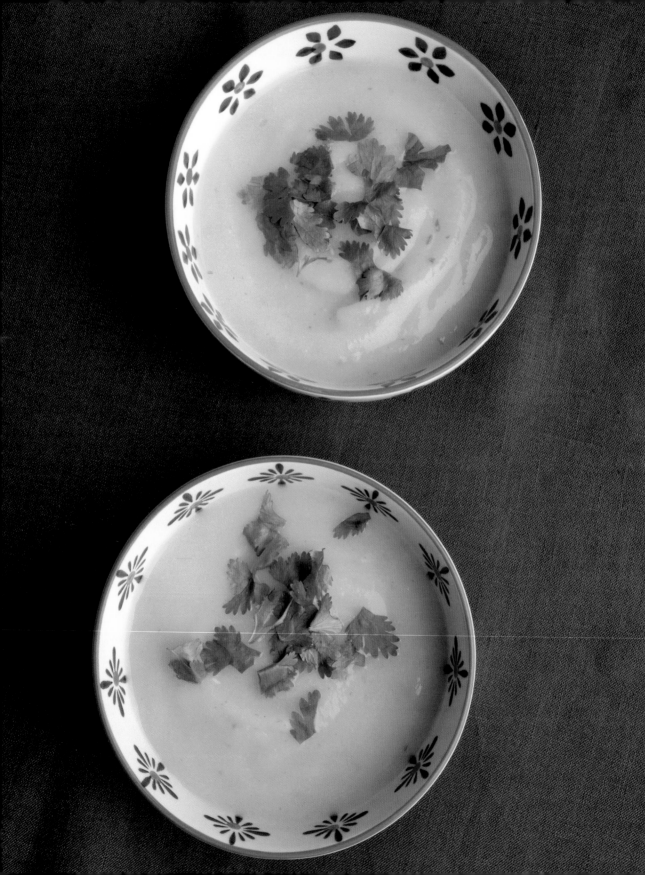

Curried Cauliflower and Potato Soup

Meal: Main, Soup

Main Ingredients:
Cauliflower, Potatoes

Prep Time: 25 minutes
plus marinating

Cook Time: 50 minutes

SERVES 4 TO 6

HEALTH CONSIDERATIONS: IN TREATMENT; GLUTEN-FREE; HIGH FIBER; HEALTHY SURVIVORSHIP; NEUTROPENIC DIET

FOOD PREFERENCE: VEGETARIAN

Cauliflower is a star of the cruciferous vegetable family but it can be bland. That's not the case for this smooth, mild soup inspired by the classic pairing of cauliflower and potatoes found in Northern Indian cooking. The cauliflower is deliciously and delicately spicy, and because there's no cayenne pepper in the spice mix, a terrific example of how spices can bring wonderful flavor without heat. If you'd like a little kick of heat, however, all you have to do is add a quarter teaspoon of ground cayenne, or to taste, to the ground spices and you're off.

1 head cauliflower broken into ½-inch florets, greens and hard core discarded

2 tablespoons ghee, canola, or grapeseed oil

1 teaspoon whole cumin seeds

3 cloves garlic, peeled and sliced

1 medium yellow onion, diced

1 teaspoon grated lemon zest

Sea salt, to taste

1 large or 2 medium Idaho or russet potatoes (about 12 ounces), scrubbed and cut into 1-inch dice

1 teaspoon ground cumin

2 teaspoons ground coriander

½ teaspoon turmeric

¼ teaspoon cayenne (optional)

¼ cup full-fat or 2% plain yogurt (see Ann's Tips, below)

6 cups stock or water

Juice of ½ lemon

Chopped cilantro, to garnish

1. Soak the cauliflower florets in cold water for 30 minutes. Drain.
2. While the cauliflower is soaking, heat the oil in a Dutch oven over medium-high heat. When the oil is hot, add the cumin seeds and let the oil sizzle a few seconds until it darkens and gives off a toasty aroma. Add the garlic and stir. As soon as the garlic colors, add the onion and lemon zest. Sprinkle with salt and sauté, about 2 minutes, until the onion starts to soften. Add the potatoes and mix well. Sprinkle with salt, and sweat partially covered for 5 to 8 minutes, or until the onion is soft and translucent.
3. Add the ground cumin, coriander, turmeric, and cayenne, if using, to the vegetables and cook, stirring to coat, for 1 minute. Add the yogurt and mix into the vegetables and spices. Cook the yogurt down until all the liquid has boiled away and just the curds remain. Add the drained cauliflower and sauté until it is covered with spices and yogurt. Add the stock, mix well, bring to a boil, then lower the heat. Cover and simmer for 30 minutes or until both the cauliflower and potatoes are very soft.
4. Turn off the heat and stir in the lemon juice. Check for salt. Let the soup sit 5 minutes. Blend in the pot with an immersion blender or in an upright blender until smooth. Serve generously sprinkled with chopped cilantro.

Ann's Tips

· 🎋 ·

Don't use fat-free plain yogurt for this recipe; it requires the thickness and fat content of at least 2% yogurt to achieve the right taste and texture.

Use caution when blending hot liquids in an upright blender (see page 11).

If you are on a neutropenic diet, microwave your soup after adding the cilantro garnish, or add the garnish to the soup and cook for 3 minutes or nuke your garnished portion in the microwave.

Non-vegetarians can make this with chicken stock. See page 24 for homemade.

Japanese Curry Noodle Soup

HEALTH CONSIDERATIONS: IN TREATMENT; HEALTHY SURVIVORSHIP; NEUTROPENIC DIET

FOOD PREFERENCE: DAIRY-FREE

Meal: Main, Soup

Main Ingredient: Noodles

Prep Time: 20 minutes

Cook Time: 30 minutes

SERVES 4

This low-heat spicy soup is both warming and soothing to sip on during treatment. It's super simple to make but uses three pots—we promise the taste is worth it if you're up to it, but see Ann's Tips, next page, for a quicker version. You don't have to trawl all over town to find Japanese curry; this will taste right made with any mild curry powder. Traditionally the soup should be quite thick, so add only just enough hot broth to cover the noodles before adding the curry sauce, and add more to taste.

2 to 3 teaspoons mild curry powder

5 cups hot Quick, Rich Chicken Broth (page 24) or Basic Vegetable Broth (page 21), divided

1 tablespoon grated ginger

1 teaspoon honey

Sea salt, to taste

½ pound skinless chicken breast, cut into ½-inch dice (see Ann's Tips, next page)

1 tablespoon cornstarch

2 tablespoons grapeseed oil

1 medium onion, thinly sliced

2 large Yukon Gold potatoes, cut into ½-inch dice

2 large carrots, peeled and cut into ½-inch dice

2 whole scallions, thinly sliced

8 ounces soba or udon noodles, cooked and drained

1. In a small bowl, mix the curry powder with 1 to 2 tablespoons of the broth and blend into a loose paste. Mix in the grated ginger, honey, and a pinch of salt. Set aside.

2. Toss the chicken together with the cornstarch until thinly coated. Set aside. Discard any remaining cornstarch.

3. Heat the oil in a wide Dutch oven over medium-high heat. Add the chicken and brown, 3 to 5 minutes. Add the vegetables, sprinkle with salt, and sauté until the onion starts to wilt. Cover, lower the heat to medium-low, and gently cook the vegetables for 8 minutes or until they are almost soft, stirring from time to time.

4. Add the curry paste and cook for 1 minute, then add ½ cup of the broth. Raise the heat to bring the soup to a low simmer. Cook until a thick sauce forms and the vegetables are tender, about 15 minutes. Add a little broth if the sauce gets too thick.

5. Bring the remaining broth to a boil. Taste for salt and add the scallions. Cook for 2 minutes. Divide the noodles among 4 bowls. Ladle the hot stock over the noodles, just enough to cover, then ladle the chicken and vegetable curry on top of the noodles. Eat immediately.

Ann's Tips

· 🦋 ·

For a vegetarian version, substitute firm tofu cut into ½-inch dice for the chicken and add it in step 4 after you've added the broth and brought the curry to a simmer. To add the cornstarch: At the end of step 3, sprinkle the cornstarch over the vegetables and stir in to mix. Cook 30 seconds, then add the curry paste.

For speed and ease, in step 5, mix 4 cups of broth directly into the curry sauce and bring to a boil. It's not traditional, but it saves a pan. And instead of using dried soba or udon noodles, use either packaged soft udon noodles that can be microwaved, or Thai rice sticks that just need covering with hot water until they soften. This will save you a pot to wash.

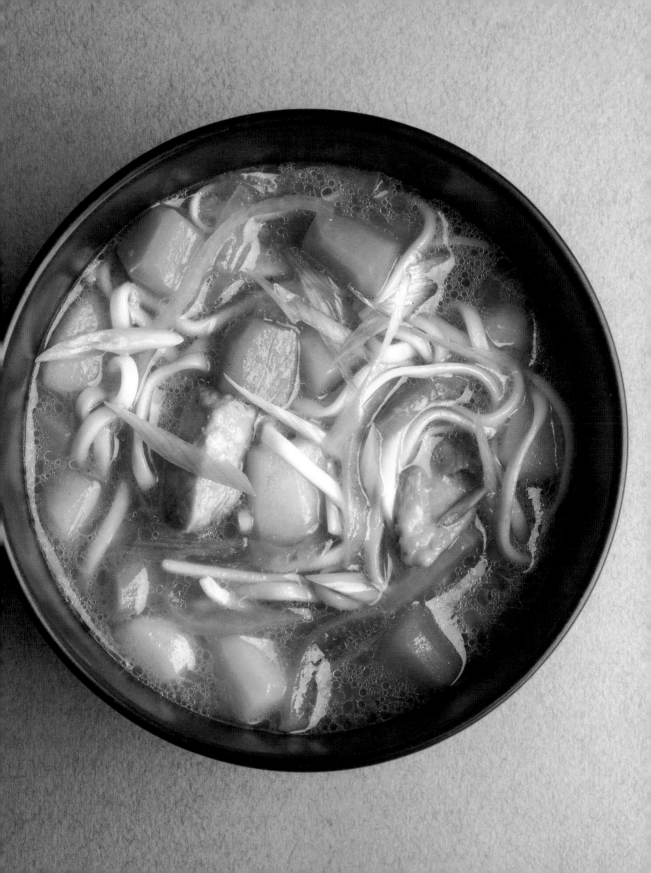

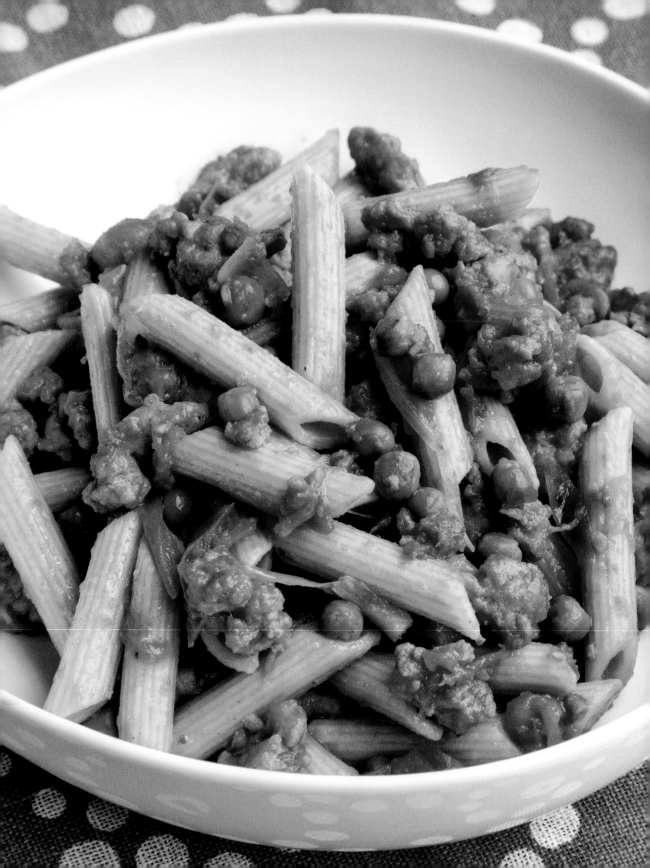

Pasta with Chicken Sausage and Peas

Meal: Main

Main Ingredients: Pasta, Chicken sausage

Prep Time: 15 minutes

Cook Time: 25 minutes

SERVES 4

HEALTH CONSIDERATIONS: IN TREATMENT; FATIGUE; NEUTROPENIC DIET

FOOD PREFERENCE: NONE

Pasta has to be one of the quickest, most satisfying meals to throw together when time is short or energy is low. This quick and easy pasta dish is another favorite from my kitchen. If you start making the sauce when you put the pasta water on to boil, it will be ready by the time the pasta is cooked. I always keep chicken sausage in the freezer as a standby for pasta, and everything else in the recipe is pretty much a pantry item, right down to the lemon. Freshly grated Parmesan is an amazing flavor enhancer. It is added here not to make the sauce cheesy but to add taste instead of salt, and boy does it!

8 ounces whole-wheat penne, rigatoni, or any other chunky pasta

2 tablespoons extra-virgin olive oil

1 teaspoon fennel seeds

1 teaspoon lemon zest

2 cloves garlic, peeled, smashed, and thinly sliced

3 Italian-style sweet chicken sausages squeezed out of their casings (see Ann's Tips, next page)

1 medium shallot, peeled, halved, and thinly sliced

1 small dried red chili pepper, deseeded and broken into small pieces (optional)

Sea salt and freshly ground black pepper, to taste

Juice of ½ lemon

1 (14-ounce) can crushed tomatoes

1 to 2 tablespoons freshly grated Parmesan cheese, plus extra for garnish

1 cup frozen peas, or to taste

1. Put water on for the pasta to boil. Cook the pasta 1 minute less than the package directions suggest. Reserve 1 cup of the cooking water, drain, and set aside.

2. Meanwhile, heat the oil in a heavy frying pan at medium-high heat. Add the fennel, lemon zest, and garlic. Cook for 1 minute, or until the garlic starts to become fragrant, then add the sausage, flattening and breaking it up into small pieces as you fry, until all the pink has gone and it starts to brown, about 5 minutes.

3. Add the shallot and the hot pepper, if using. Sprinkle with salt and sauté until the shallot starts to take color and caramelize, 3 to 5 minutes. Deglaze the pan with the lemon juice and add the tomatoes. Sprinkle with salt and lower the heat to a simmer. Cook the sauce until the tomatoes look saucy and syrupy, 5 to 8 minutes.

4. Check the sauce. Add some of the reserved pasta water if it looks too dry. Stir in the Parmesan and when it has melted into the sauce, stir in the peas. Check for salt.

5. Add the pasta to the sausage mixture in the pan with more of the reserved water to taste. Turn to mix well and coat the pasta in the sauce. Cook 1 minute more over medium-high heat or until the pasta is coated and al dente. Grind some black pepper over the pan and serve with more grated Parmesan cheese.

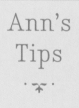

Ann's Tips

You can also use hot Italian-style chicken sausage for this dish. If you do, unless you like really spicy food, don't add the dried pepper in step 3.

Vietnamese-Style Noodle Salad with Grilled Chicken

Meal: Main

Main Ingredients:
Chicken, Rice noodles, Cabbage

Prep Time: 30 minutes, plus 30 minutes for marinating

Cook Time: 10 minutes

SERVES 4

HEALTH CONSIDERATIONS: IN TREATMENT; HIGH FIBER; GLUTEN-FREE; HEALTHY SURVIVORSHIP

FOOD PREFERENCE: DAIRY-FREE; NUTS

This cool, light, easy noodle salad is perfect for a hot summer day. It's a sensational mix of tastes and flavors, particularly if you like spicy food, which I do, and it puts napa cabbage on the table. And if I remember to do it, to get an extra chili kick I leave the chicken in the fridge to marinate overnight.

Health Tip

For those with tree nut and peanut allergies, instead of peanuts try topping with chopped toasted pumpkin seeds or sunflower seeds.

Vietnamese-Style Dressing
3 tablespoons Thai or Vietnamese fish sauce

½ cup plus 1 tablespoon lime juice

1½ to 2 teaspoons sugar, or to taste

1 to 2 small hot serrano chilies, or to taste, very thinly sliced

1 clove garlic, peeled and smashed

Salad
2 teaspoons grapeseed or peanut oil

4 pieces thinly sliced chicken breast (escalopes)

8 ounces Thai rice sticks

1 cup thinly shredded napa cabbage

1 cup soy bean sprouts

½ cup grated carrot

2 tablespoons thinly sliced scallions

3 to 4 tablespoons chopped, dry-toasted peanuts

4 sprigs mint or Thai basil, leaves stripped and shredded

1. Make the dressing: In a medium-size bowl, whisk the fish sauce, lime juice, and sugar until well blended. Stir in the chilies. Add the garlic. Spoon 4 tablespoons of the dressing into a baking dish. Reserve the rest.

2. Into the 4 tablespoons of dressing in the dish, with a fork mix in the oil. Add the chicken pieces and spoon the dressing in the baking dish over them. Place in the fridge and allow to marinate for 30 minutes to 1 hour. Turn once. If you like your chicken spicy, add more sliced chilies to the dish.

3. While the chicken is marinating, put the rice sticks in a large bowl and completely cover with boiling water. Let them sit until they soften to al dente, about 5 minutes. Drain, then rinse with cold running water to stop them from cooking more. Distribute evenly among four bowls. Pile the vegetables on top of the noodles, with the cabbage and bean sprouts first, then the carrot. Set aside while you cook the chicken.

4. Heat a grill pan over medium-high heat. When it is hot, grill the chicken for 5 minutes on each side or until it is browned and cooked through. If the slices are very thin, this may be quicker than the time given. Remove from the grill and thinly slice into diagonal strips.

5. To serve: Top the bowls with the chicken slices and spoon the reserved dressing over them. Sprinkle with the scallions and the peanuts. Serve with a generous garnish of basil or mint leaves.

Ann's Tips

· ⅄ ·

For a really spicy dressing, use red Thai bird chilies. Spicy-hot chilies are rich in capsaicin, which is analgesic and anti-inflammatory. Science aside, I find them quite addictive. Analgesic or not, be very careful after cutting hot chilies. Their oils get everywhere and won't wash off your hands straightaway, so don't touch your eyes, nose, or other sensitive areas of your body after handling them or you could be in for an unwanted and unpleasant surprise.

To make this family-style, put the noodles, vegetables, and grilled chicken in a large bowl. Toss with the toppings, herbs, and Vietnamese dressing. Serve.

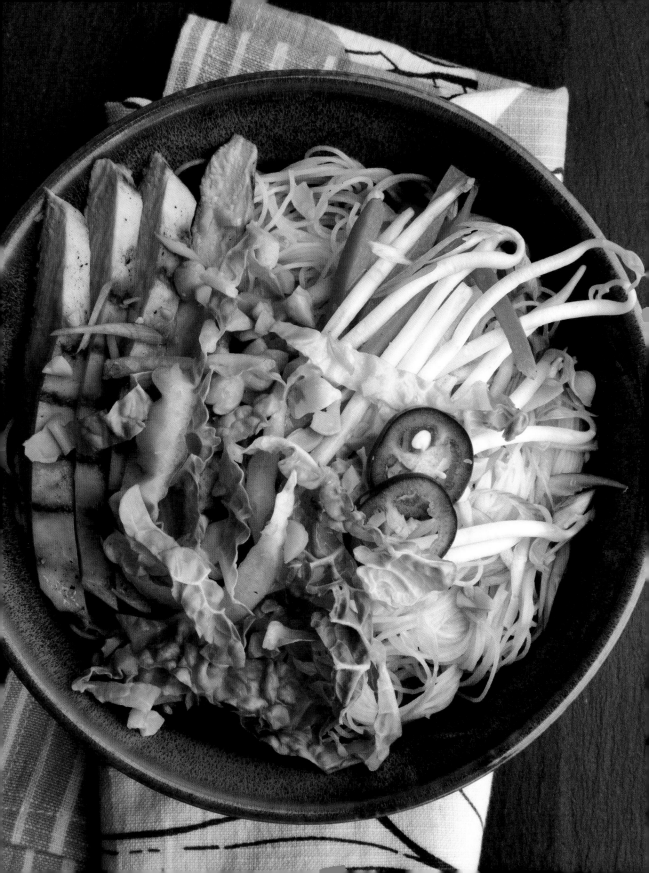

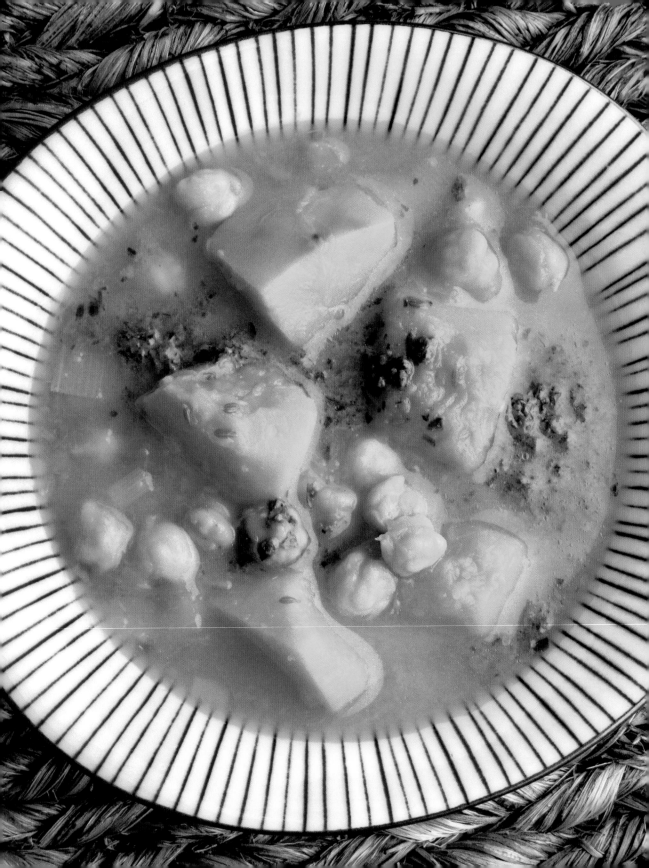

Moroccan Pumpkin Stew with Chermoula Sauce

Meal: Main

Main Ingredient:
Kabocha squash

Prep Time: 30 minutes

Cook Time: 50 minutes

SERVES 6 TO 8

HEALTH CONSIDERATIONS: IN TREATMENT; EASY TO SWALLOW (SEE ANN'S TIPS, NEXT PAGE); GLUTEN-FREE; HIGH FIBER; HEALTHY SURVIVORSHIP; NEUTROPENIC DIET

FOOD PREFERENCE: DAIRY-FREE; VEGAN; VEGETARIAN

This easy dish with a smoky back taste is a wonderful antidote to a chilly winter's day, especially when livened up by the bright flavors of chermoula sauce. Chermoula is a basic of Moroccan cooking and the granddaddy of the salsa verde used in Hispanic cooking. It works wonderfully with sweet winter squash in this stew. I love the soft, starchy texture of kabocha, but if you can't find it, don't fret; butternut will do the job. Better yet, butternut squash can often be found peeled and precut, a huge energy saver if treatment has left you tired.

1 dried chipotle pepper, whole

4 cups water, divided

2 tablespoons extra-virgin olive oil

1 teaspoon cumin seeds

2 leeks, white parts only, diced

1 bay leaf

1 (2-pound) kabocha or butternut squash, peeled, deseeded, and cut into 1-inch dice

Sea salt, to taste

1 (14-ounce) can chickpeas, drained and rinsed (see Ann's Tips, next page)

Chermoula Sauce

2 cloves garlic, peeled, smashed, and chopped

¼ cup extra-virgin olive oil

1 teaspoon ground cumin

¼ teaspoon hot paprika

Juice of 1 large lemon

⅔ cup coarsely chopped cilantro

⅓ cup coarsely chopped parsley

Sea salt, to taste

1. Cover the chipotle pepper in 1 cup of boiling water and let it soak for 30 minutes. Remove the pepper and set aside, reserving the soaking water.

2. Heat the oil in a Dutch oven over medium-high heat. Add the cumin seeds and let them sizzle for a minute, then add the leeks and bay leaf. Cook until they start to soften. Add the kabocha and the soaked chipotle pepper, and sprinkle the vegetables with salt. Lower the heat and allow to sweat, partially covered, for 10 minutes. The kabocha will start to soften.

3. Add the reserved chipotle soaking water and enough water to just cover the vegetables. Bring to a boil over high heat. Cover, reduce the heat to medium-low, and simmer for 20 minutes. Add the chickpeas. If the stew looks slightly dry, add a little of the remaining water. Continue cooking until the squash can be mashed against the sides of the pan, 15 to 20 minutes. Turn off the heat and let the soup sit for 10 minutes.

4. Meanwhile, make the chermoula sauce: In a blender or small food processor, process together the garlic, oil, spices, and lemon juice at high speed until they are well blended with no lumps of raw garlic. Add the green herbs and the salt. Blend until you have a tan sauce flecked with green.

5. Taste the soup for salt. Discard the chipotle, and ladle the stew into individual bowls. Serve with a teaspoonful of the chermoula sauce stirred into each.

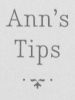

Ann's Tips

Chermoula sauce is a great addition to all kinds of dishes. Bag and freeze any leftovers.

Although canned beans are convenient, homemade chickpeas are delicious. They freeze well, too. For this recipe, you can use 2 cups of cooked Spicy Chickpeas in Chipotle Broth (page 37). If you do, you won't need the chipotle pepper—the heat and flavor are in the chickpeas already—and in step 2 add only 2 to 3 cups of liquid since you'll be using the chickpea broth as well.

If you need something easy to swallow, when the stew is cooked, discard the chipotle pepper and bay leaf and blend the stew in a blender at high speed for a thick, smooth soup. Drizzle with chermoula, if desired, or top with plain yogurt.

Curried Eggplant in Peanut Sauce

Meal: Main

Main Ingredients:
Eggplant, Peanuts, Coconut

Prep Time: 30 minutes

Cook Ttime: 45 minutes

SERVES 4

HEALTH CONSIDERATIONS: IN TREATMENT; HIGH FIBER; GLUTEN-FREE; NEUTROPENIC DIET; HEALTHY SURVIVORSHIP

FOOD PREFERENCE: DAIRY-FREE; VEGAN; VEGETARIAN; NUTS

Using spices is one of the things we are always asked about at classes, and with good reason: Spices like turmeric have cancer-fighting anti-oxidant properties that come out best when cooked, but classic American cooking doesn't use them that much. In my opinion, South Asian cooking, the spice powerhouse, knows how to do it best. This easy, tasty curry is a great example. It has only four ingredients that actually need prepping—the eggplant, onion, and tomato, plus a hit of freshly grated ginger to finish the dish. Everything else comes out of a can or spice jar. To my mind, when cooking with spices the trick is to start by measuring out all the spices for your recipe to keep by the stove for easy access. After that, it's easy.

2 teaspoons mustard seeds

½ teaspoon cumin seeds

½ teaspoon turmeric

½ teaspoon cayenne, or to taste

6 to 8 baby or fairy eggplants (see Ann's Tips, next page)

2 to 3 tablespoons coconut oil (3 to 4 tablespoons if using Italian eggplant)

1 red onion, peeled, halved, and thinly sliced

1 teaspoon sea salt, or to taste

1 cup chopped beefsteak tomato (about 1 large tomato)

2 tablespoons unsweetened smooth peanut butter

4 ounces coconut milk (about ½ cup) (see Ann's Tips, next page) plus ¼ cup water

1 to 2 teaspoons freshly grated gingerroot

1. Measure out the spices and set by the stove.
2. Trim the stalk ends from the eggplants and cut 4 shallow slits in the skin lengthwise. This will allow the eggplants to expand as they cook.
3. Heat the coconut oil in a large Dutch oven over medium-high heat. Fry the eggplants until browned and puffed up, 8 to 10 minutes. Remove with tongs and set aside.
4. To the same oil add the mustard seeds. Let them cook for a minute over medium-high heat. Use a spatter guard over the pan, as the mustard seeds will pop in the hot oil. Quickly add the cumin seeds, cook for 30 seconds, then add the onion and sprinkle with salt. Fry until soft and golden, about 8 minutes.
5. Add the turmeric and cayenne to the onion. Cook for 1 minute. Add the tomato. Cook until it starts to soften, about 5 minutes. Stir in the peanut butter until blended, then add the coconut milk mixture. Return the eggplant to the sauce. Lower the heat to medium-low and cook, stirring occasionally, until the sauce has thickened, about 20 minutes. Add a little water if it looks too thick.
6. Add the ginger. Cook for 2 minutes more. Turn off the heat. Let it sit for 5 to 10 minutes for the flavor to develop. Check for salt. Serve with boiled basmati rice.

Ann's Tips

· ✈ ·

If you can't find the tiny fairy eggplants, it's okay to use a larger variety. Use 2 to 3 medium-size fruits of a skinny Asian eggplant variety. Cut them in half lengthwise and then into 1-inch pieces. If they are very slender, just cut them into 1-inch pieces. You can also use 1 medium black Italian eggplant cut into 1-inch cubes.

To keep the eggplant from soaking up too much oil, toss it with 2 tablespoons of the coconut oil and roast it on a parchment-lined baking sheet in the upper third of a 425°F oven for 15 minutes, turning halfway through.

If you can find only the 14-ounce cans of coconut milk, stir it well, take what the recipe needs, and freeze the rest in a ziplock bag, where it will keep for 3 to 4 months.

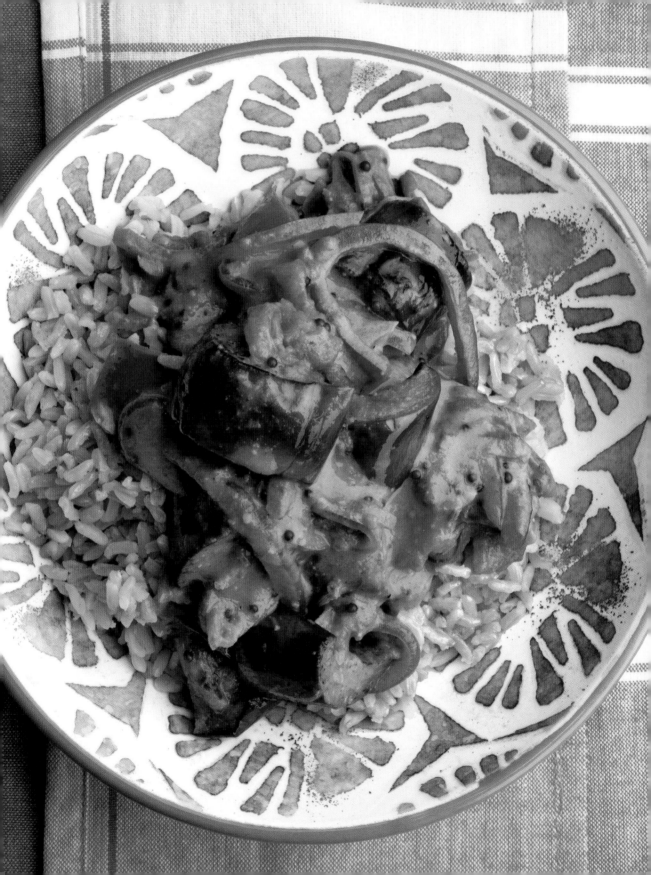

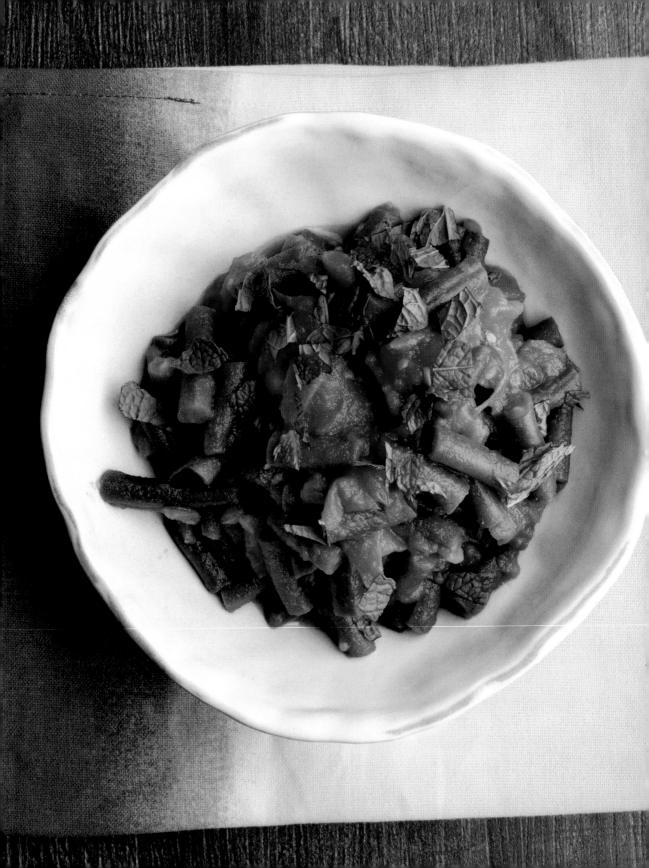

Spiced Green Beans with Tomatoes

Meal: Side

Main Ingredients: Green beans, Tomatoes

Prep Time: 30 minutes

Cook Time: 25 minutes

SERVES 4

HEALTH CONSIDERATIONS: IN TREATMENT; FATIGUE; HIGH FIBER; GLUTEN-FREE; NEUTROPENIC DIET; HEALTHY SURVIVORSHIP

FOOD PREFERENCE: DAIRY-FREE; VEGAN; VEGETARIAN

I love these beans. They are an easy one-pot dish and a great way to tastily change up fresh or frozen green beans as a side for simply cooked chicken, fish, or tofu. I even like them on their own with brown rice. They have a mildly spicy flavor, but if you want to up the ante and add some heat, stir in the optional cayenne.

2 tablespoons extra-virgin olive oil

1 teaspoon cumin seeds

1 (½-inch) piece gingerroot, cut into thin julienne

1 clove garlic, thinly sliced

2 medium shallots, thinly sliced

Sea salt, to taste

3 cups green beans, trimmed and cut into 1-inch pieces (see Ann's Tips, next page)

½ teaspoon turmeric

½ teaspoon cayenne (optional, and to taste)

1 cup quartered cherry tomatoes (see Ann's Tips, next page)

Juice of ½ lemon

2 tablespoons chopped mint

1. Heat the oil in a wok or sauté pan with a lid over medium-high heat. When the oil starts to shimmer, add the cumin. Let the cumin sizzle for 30 seconds, then add the ginger and garlic. When the garlic starts to color slightly, add the shallots, sprinkle with salt, and cook, stirring, until they soften and start to color, about 3 minutes.
2. Add the green beans and cook, stirring, until the shallots have started to brown

and the beans have turned a bright green, about 3 minutes. Sprinkle with the turmeric and cayenne, if using, and stir to mix. Cook for 1 minute more.

3. Add the chopped tomatoes. Sauté for 2 minutes, scraping any bits from the bottom of the pan into the sauce. Sprinkle with salt. Cover, reduce the heat to medium-low, and cook for 10 to 15 minutes, or until the beans are just soft. Taste for salt. Stir in the lemon juice and chopped mint, and cook for 30 seconds. Serve immediately.

Ann's Tips

You can also use frozen green beans. Instead of adding them in step 2, add them in step 3, after the tomatoes have been cooking for 5 to 8 minutes. Stir them in still frozen, and cook for an extra 3 to 5 minutes, until just cooked.

In the summer, when tomatoes are at their best, dice up some Roma or beefsteak tomatoes to make this dish. In the winter, you can also use canned tomatoes in place of the cherry tomatoes.

Spicy Spinach with Lentils

HEALTH CONSIDERATIONS: IN TREATMENT; HIGH FIBER; FATIGUE; GLUTEN-FREE; HEALTHY SURVIVORSHIP; NEUTROPENIC DIET

FOOD PREFERENCE: DAIRY-FREE; VEGAN; VEGETARIAN

Meal: Side, Main

Main Ingredients:
Spinach, Lentils

Prep Time: 30 minutes

Cook Time: 35 minutes

SERVES 4

This lightly spicy dish is an easy way to get some South Asian flavor. Eat it with some brown rice and you'll have an easy, protein-packed dinner. Look for the smaller brown lentils, instead of the large flat green ones. They hold their shape better. Green lentils can break up suddenly if they overcook even a little, and for this it's nice if the lentils stay whole. In any event, to be on the safe side, test the lentils after they've been cooking for 30 minutes to see if they are done. And if you can find garam marsala spice mix, be sure to try it.

1 cup brown lentils, picked through and washed

3 to 4 cups water

6 cloves garlic, peeled and smashed, divided

Sea salt, to taste

2 tablespoons extra-virgin olive oil

6 to 8 whole cloves (see Ann's Tips, next page)

3 jalapeño peppers, or to taste, deseeded and sliced

1 small shallot, thinly sliced

1 large ripe beefsteak tomato, diced (see Ann's Tips, next page)

1 pound baby spinach (see Ann's Tips, next page)

¼ teaspoon garam masala (optional)

4 lemon wedges

1. Combine the lentils, 3 cups of water, 4 of the garlic cloves, and a generous pinch of salt in a heavy 2- or 3-quart pot. Bring to a boil, reduce the heat to medium-low, and cook for 30 to 35 minutes, or until the lentils are just soft but not mushy. If the lentils look dry during cooking, add the remaining water, a little at a time. Drain.

2. While the lentils are cooking, chop the remaining garlic. Heat the oil in a sauté

pan over medium-high heat. Add the cloves, and when they start to swell and pop, add the remaining garlic and jalapeños. Cook, stirring, until the garlic starts to color, about 1 minute.

3. Add the shallot and cook about 5 minutes, or until it turns translucent. Add the diced tomato and sprinkle with salt. Cook until they start to soften and look saucy, about 5 minutes. Discard the whole cloves (see Ann's Tips, below).

4. Add the spinach in batches, mixing it in as you go. As soon as the first batch wilts, add another. Continue until all the spinach has been added in.

5. Stir in the lentils and cook for 2 to 3 minutes. Taste for salt. Sprinkle with garam masala, if using, and stir in. Serve as a side with lemon wedges or over rice for a simple supper.

Ann's Tips

· ⚕ ·

A 10-ounce box of frozen leaf spinach will do nicely to make this dish. Just thaw it and press out any excess water before adding it to the tomato and spices. You also can use bunched spinach; 2 bunches will do it for this dish, but fresh spinach is time-consuming to wash and prepare properly.

If you use powdered cloves, ⅓ teaspoon will do. Add it in step 2 just as the shallots take color, cook for 1 minute, then add the tomato.

Speaking of tomato, in the winter when fresh tomatoes aren't that good, either use 1 cup of quartered cherry tomatoes, or ¾ to 1 cup of canned diced tomatoes. You can freeze the leftovers.

If you can't find the cloves after cooking, don't worry, they soften as they cook and will not overwhelm the dish with seasoning.

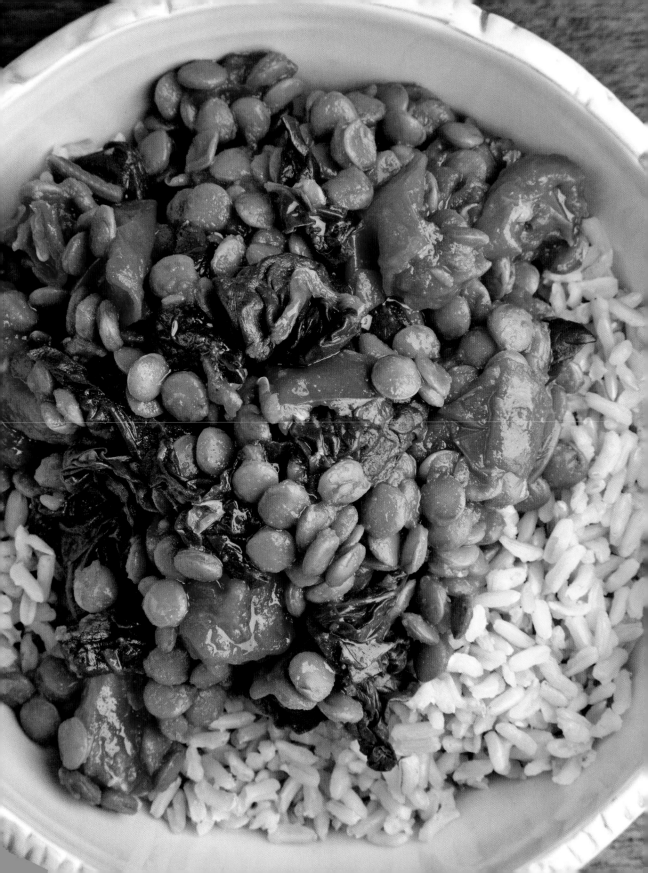

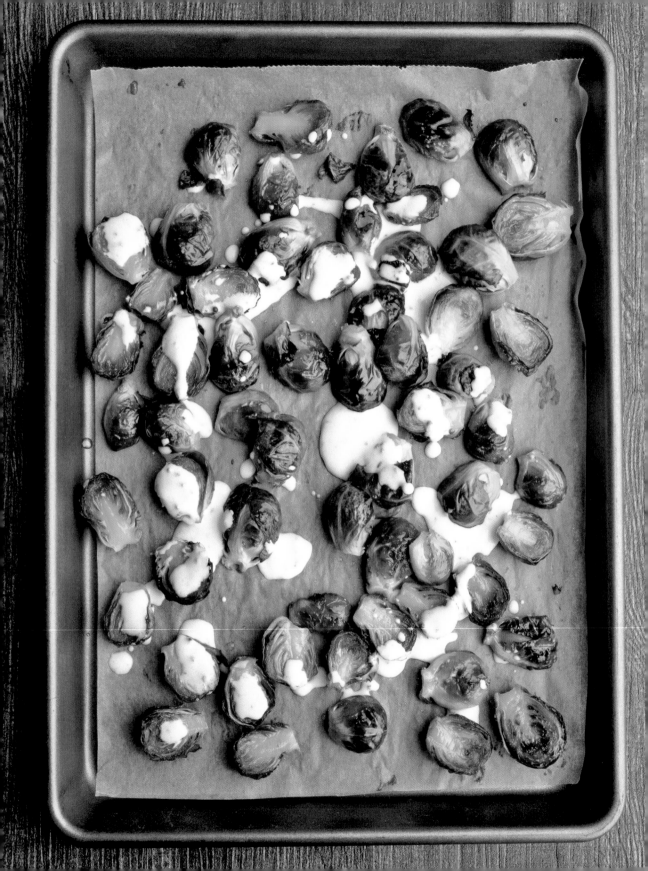

Roasted Brussels Sprouts with Spiced Yogurt Sauce

Meal: Side; Basics, Sauces

Main Ingredients: Brussels sprouts, Yogurt

Prep Time: 10 to 15 minutes

Cook Time: 8 minutes

SERVES 4 TO 6

HEALTH CONSIDERATIONS: IN TREATMENT; GLUTEN-FREE; HIGH FIBER; HEALTHY SURVIVORSHIP; NEUTROPENIC DIET

FOOD PREFERENCE: VEGETARIAN

This is a simple, delicious side dish that makes the most of some fabulously healthy ingredients: the cruciferous powerhouse, brussels sprouts, topped with a spicily probiotic yogurt sauce. As both are delicious in their own right, eat them separately or together. Try the sauce on burgers, veggies, or as a cooling condiment to curries. You won't be disappointed.

Health Tip

If you are on a neutropenic diet, check to see how your doctor feels about eating probiotics like yogurt before chowing down on the sauce.

Brussels Sprouts

1 pound brussels sprouts, trimmed and halved

2 tablespoons extra-virgin olive oil

Sea salt and freshly ground pepper, to taste

Spiced Yogurt Sauce

1 teaspoon extra-virgin olive oil

1 clove garlic, minced

2 teaspoons cumin seeds

2 teaspoons fennel seeds

1 teaspoon mustard seeds

1⅓ cups plain yogurt (see Ann's Tips, next page)

Zest and juice of 1 lemon

1. Preheat the broiler. Line a baking sheet with aluminum foil and set aside.
2. Toss the brussels sprouts with oil, salt, and pepper. Spread in one even layer on the prepared baking sheet. Place under the broiler on a center rung and broil for 8 minutes, or until the sprouts can be pierced with a fork and are a little golden-flecked with dark spots. Turn them halfway through to ensure even cooking.
3. Meanwhile, make the sauce: In a small skillet, heat 1 teaspoon of oil over medium-high heat. Add the garlic, cumin, fennel seeds, and mustard seeds. Cook for about 1 minute, or until the mustard seeds pop. Remove from the heat and smash the mixture with a mortar and pestle or chop finely on a cutting board. Stir into the yogurt with the salt, lemon zest, and lemon juice. Taste for seasoning.
4. Serve the brussels sprouts on a platter with yogurt spooned over them or as a dipping sauce on the side.

Ann's Tips

· ✶ ·

Use either whole or 2% milk plain yogurt for the sauce, not fat-free. This sauce needs some fat. For a thicker consistency, use Greek yogurt.

Honeydew Melon and Ginger Lassi

Meal: Beverage, Snack, Breakfast

Main Ingredient: Melon

Prep Time: 10 minutes

SERVES 6

HEALTH CONSIDERATIONS: IN TREATMENT; FATIGUE; EASY TO SWALLOW; NAUSEA; BLAND DIET; LOW FIBER; GLUTEN-FREE; HEALTHY SURVIVORSHIP

FOOD PREFERENCE: VEGETARIAN

Creamy, delicious lassi is the Indian way to drink yogurt. It is a refreshing taste sensation. I've suggested using honey or agave because spoon for spoon, both are twice as sweet as sugar. If you use honey, particularly Medihoney Manuka or raw organic honey, you will not only get more sweetness for your calories, you can enjoy its reputed medicinal properties, too. Ginger is no slouch, either. Aside from tasting good, it aids digestion and cools the body.

1½ cups diced honeydew melon, chilled

1 tablespoon fresh lemon juice

1 tablespoon chopped ginger

1 teaspoon honey or agave nectar

¼ cup plain Greek yogurt

1. Put all the ingredients in a blender and blend until smooth. Serve over ice.

Ann's Tips

For more of a classic smoothie texture, add an extra ½ cup of melon and 3 ice cubes.

If your mouth is sore, add 1 teaspoon grated lemon zest instead of acidic lemon juice.

Sweet

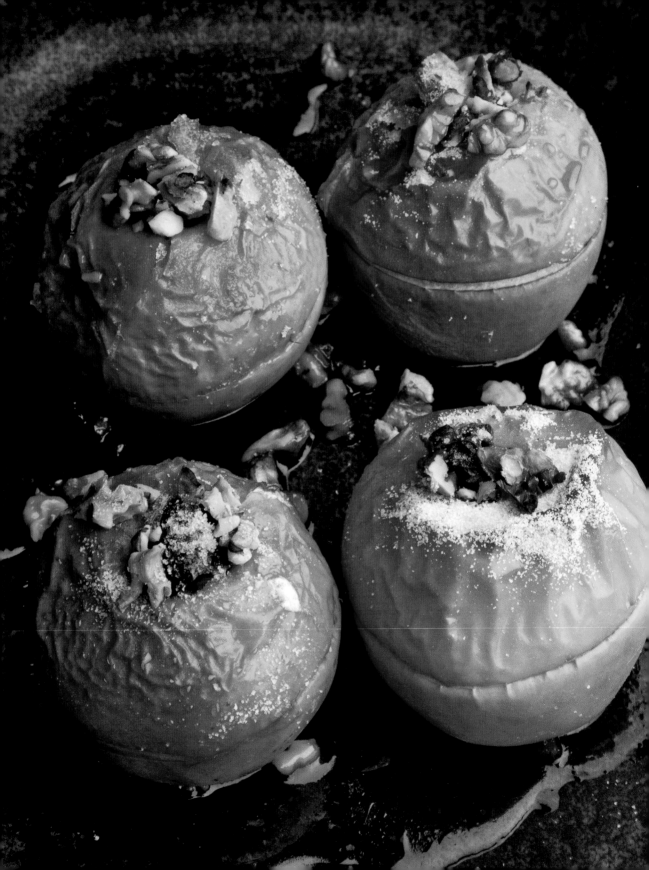

· · · · · 🦋 · · · · ·

There were always bags of cookies or boxes of doughnut holes in the chemo suite when I went for my infusions. They were supplied by both the patients and the oncology nurses. It was rare not to find sweets on the counter. A lot of people are horrified when I tell them this. And I have to admit I was, too, at first. How unhealthy! Then I understood why they were needed. It's obvious, really. Cancer treatment is bad news. Sweet treats help to mitigate a bad situation. And they're practical in their way. After an intravenous drip of Benadryl, I for one needed a little sugar to perk me up.

I have no qualms admitting I enjoyed my sweet treats while I was on chemo. During my radiation treatment, too, as it ground on, I admit the sweet treats found their way back into my pantry again. Acquiring a sweet tooth is common during treatment. I especially liked to have sweets on hand for the days after my infusions, when I was tremendously incapacitated by fatigue, and often felt achy, queasy, or nauseous. Nibbling on something sweet would help the queasiness subside and give me a little spurt of energy to get up and about, "nibbling" being the operative word here. I like to know what I'm eating, so on my more energetic days, I baked. I find baking relaxing. You get an almost instant result for your labor while doing something that keeps your mind busy, which is helpful when all you have is more chemo and radiation to look forward to. Cookies are quick and easy to make even if you're fatigued, and the more basic cakes and desserts don't require too much thought or energy to put together, either.

I've put together some of my favorite sweet ideas for you to try that are as healthy as these things can be. The recipes use whole-wheat and almond flours, and a lot less sugar than usual. But they're still treats. Once they're out of the oven, don't eat the whole batch, however tempting. It's that little bit of sweetness that will do your soul the most good.

SUGAR AND CANCER

There's a lot of talk about sugar feeding cancer cells. In one sense it's true; all our cells rely on glucose for nourishment, the cancerous and the healthy alike, but it's untrue as an absolute statement. All the food we eat ends up in our blood as glucose and is used by all our cells to give our bodies energy. Sugars and refined carbs just get there faster than whole foods, giving us those peaks and valleys of the sugar high. The difficulty with sugar is that it's used in almost every package of processed food we eat and it's this overuse that gives all sugar a bad rap. I believe that an occasional bit of sweetness is okay. Our brains need it, but you should eat sugar knowingly.

STORING THE GOODIES

When baking cakes and cookies, it's useful to have an airtight tin to store them in, like those old-fashioned cookie tins. Lined with some wax paper, they keep cookies and cakes incredibly well. Cookie dough can be frozen, and some of the simple loaf cakes like pound cake and banana bread will freeze well, too, and are good toasted, so slice them up, and bag and freeze them for later.

Honeyed Pistachio Cookies

HEALTH CONSIDERATIONS: IN TREATMENT; NAUSEA; NEUTROPENIC DIET

FOOD PREFERENCE: VEGETARIAN; NUTS

Ambrosial is a word that could be used to describe these heavenly little cookies. Inspired by the honeyed sweets found around the eastern end of the Mediterranean, these cookies are incredibly easy to make and a real treat for patients and caregivers alike. Pistachios are heart-healthy and have antioxidant properties. But although they bring benefits to the table, don't forget they're part of a honey cookie, and all sweets should be eaten in moderation. They are naughty but nice!

Meal: Dessert

Main Ingredients: Pistachios, Honey

Prep Time: 25 minutes, plus 60 minutes for chilling

Cook Time: 15 minutes

MAKES 32 COOKIES

1 cup softened butter

½ cup organic granulated cane sugar

2 teaspoons vanilla extract

2½ cups all-purpose or whole-wheat pastry flour

1½ cups finely chopped shelled unsalted pistachios

⅓ cup whole-milk plain yogurt

¼ cup plus 2 tablespoons orange blossom honey or buckwheat honey, divided

1. In a large bowl, beat the butter, sugar, and vanilla together with an electric handheld mixer until creamy.
2. Add the flour and, with a pastry blender or 2 butter knives, combine the mixture until it looks crumbly. Stir in the pistachios. Add the yogurt. Mix with your fingertips until a dough is formed. Turn the dough onto a lightly floured surface and knead until well blended, about 1 minute. Wrap in wax paper or plastic wrap and chill in the refrigerator for 1 hour.
3. Preheat the oven to 350°F. Line two baking sheets with parchment paper.
4. Break off small chunks of dough and roll between your hands to form 1½-inch balls. Place them on the prepared baking sheets and flatten with the back of a fork. Take half the honey and brush the cookies generously with it, reserving

any that's left over. Bake the cookies on a middle rack in the oven for 15 minutes or until pale golden. Transfer the cookies to a wire rack on top of a sheet of wax paper.

5. While the cookies are still hot, quickly brush them with the remaining honey, adding more as the cookies absorb it until they won't take any more. Any drips will be caught on the wax paper for easy cleanup. Return any leftover honey to the jar. Cool before serving or store in an airtight tin.

Ann's Tips
· ✱ ·

To make the honey easier to handle, stand the jar in a bowl of hot water before measuring it out. It will make the honey thinner and it will brush onto the cookies more smoothly.

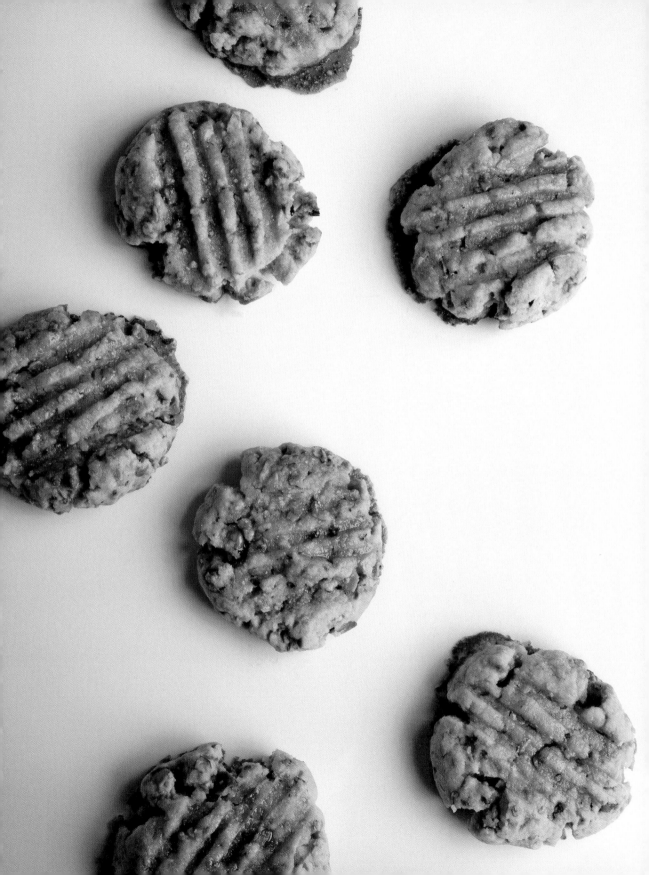

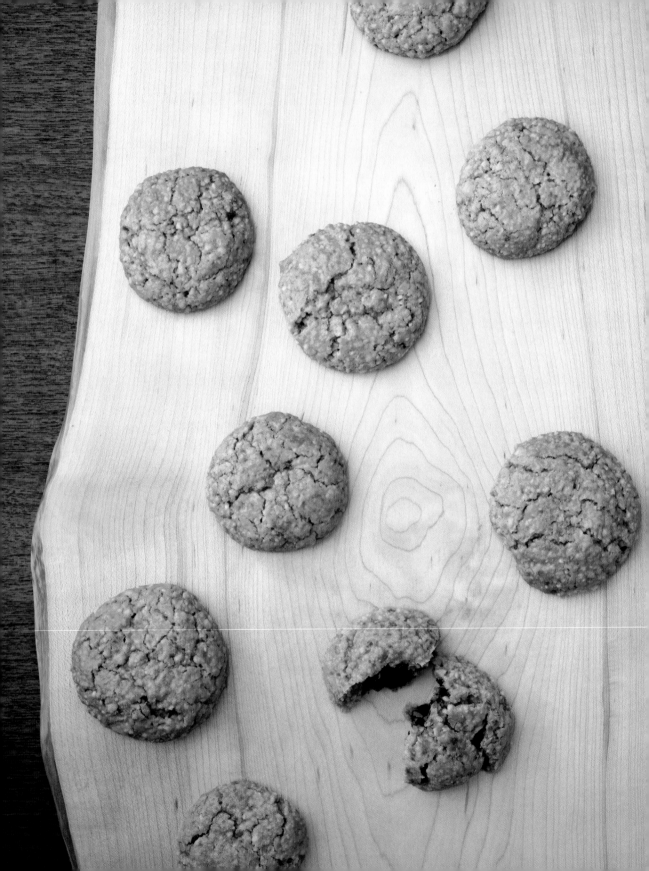

Peanut-Chocolate Cookies

HEALTH CONSIDERATIONS: IN TREATMENT; NAUSEA; GLUTEN-FREE; NEUTROPENIC DIET

FOOD PREFERENCE: VEGETARIAN; NUTS

Meal: Snack, Dessert

Main Ingredients: Peanuts, Chocolate

Prep Time: 20 minutes

Cook Time: 10 minutes

MAKES 18 TO 20 COOKIES

If peanuts and chocolate are your thing, this cookie is definitely for you. You will need a food processor to grind the nuts and sugar together, but aside from that, these yummy little delights are pretty much trouble-free. Not only do they have a chocolate surprise at their heart, they are gluten-free and high in protein. Who could ask for anything more?

3 cups roasted unsalted peanuts, loosely packed

½ cup light brown sugar

2 egg whites

Pinch of cream of tartar (optional)

1 cup confectioners' sugar (see Ann's Tips, next page)

1 (12-ounce) bag 70 percent bittersweet baking chocolate chips (see Ann's Tips, next page)

1. Preheat the oven to 325°F. Line two cookie sheets with parchment paper and set aside.
2. Add the peanuts and brown sugar to the bowl of a food processor. Pulse to the texture of fine meal. Transfer to a large mixing bowl and set aside.
3. In a separate bowl, make a meringue: Using a hand mixer, beat the egg whites together with the cream of tartar until soft peaks form. Gradually sift in the confectioners' sugar until it is completely incorporated. The egg whites will turn from stiff and dry to a thick, glossy, creamy consistency.
4. Make a well in the nut mixture and tip in the egg whites. Fold together with a rubber spatula to form a soft, sticky dough. Wet your hands and, using a tablespoon measure, scoop out a little of the dough. Depending on your taste, put 1 to 4 chocolate chips in the center, seal it in, and roll the cookie into a ball

between your hands, making sure the chocolate stays covered. Place the ball on the baking sheet and flatten the top slightly. Repeat with the remaining dough and chocolate chips. Leave space around each cookie—they will spread a little as they bake.

5. Bake on a middle rack in the oven for 10 to 12 minutes, until the cookies are pale with a few cracks on top, and lightly brown underneath.

6. Place the sheet on a cooling rack and let the cookies cool for 10 minutes. Transfer cookies directly to the cooling rack to finish cooling. Eat immediately or store in an airtight tin for up to 3 days.

Ann's Tips

· ⚘ ·

I find that these cookies come out better if baked on a baking sheet lined with parchment than with a Silpat or other silicone cookie sheets. I'm not sure why, but my guess is that it's because the parchment paper on the metal sheet distributes the heat a little differently.

Processing the peanuts in a food processor with the light brown sugar will stop them from forming a paste and keep them mealy, which is what these cookies need. A blender tends to turn them to a paste.

Egg whites rise easily if everything is very clean—they can separate if not. Adding a pinch of acidic cream of tartar to your egg whites will stabilize them, so if either your bowl or whisk is a little damp or greasy from other uses, your egg whites will still be perfect.

You can make regular granulated sugar into confectioners' sugar by pulsing it in a clean coffee grinder until it turns to powder.

I have been conservative with the amount of chocolate chips. You can add up to 6 per cookie.

Apricot and Pecan Oatmeal Cookies

Meal: Snack, Dessert

Main Ingredients: Oats, Pecans, Apricots

Prep Time: 30 minutes

Cook Time: 12 minutes

MAKES ABOUT 40 COOKIES

HEALTH CONSIDERATIONS: IN TREATMENT; FATIGUE; NAUSEA; BLAND DIET; HIGH FIBER; HIGH CALORIE; GLUTEN-FREE (SEE HEALTH TIP, BELOW); NEUTROPENIC DIET

FOOD PREFERENCE: DAIRY-FREE; VEGETARIAN

These fabulous dairy-free cookies are one of my favorites. How could they not be, loving apricots, pecans, and coconut as much as I do? They are the kind of treat that brightened my day when I was feeling low during treatment. Sweet but not cloying, they satisfied my craving for sweets with healthy ingredients, with the important dividend that they are extremely easy—indeed, almost foolproof—to make. Like most cookies, they can be made and baked in no time at all. They're on my "keepers" list.

Health Tip
These can easily be made gluten-free simply by using gluten-free flour and oats.

½ cup whole-wheat pastry flour (see Ann's Tips, next page)

1¼ cups quick-cooking oats

½ cup unsweetened shredded coconut

¾ tablespoon baking soda

½ cup chopped pecans

½ cup coconut oil, melted

¾ cup light brown sugar

1 large egg

1 teaspoon vanilla extract

½ teaspoon sea salt

½ cup chopped unsulfured dried apricots

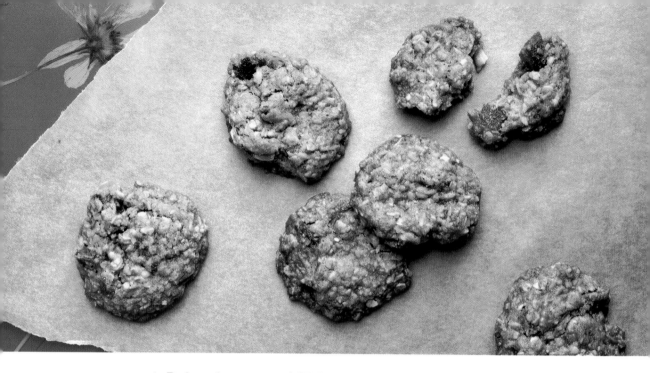

1. Preheat the oven to 350°F. Cover two large cookie sheets with parchment paper and set aside.

2. In a large bowl, stir together the flour, oats, shredded coconut, baking soda, and pecans. Make a well in the center of the bowl. Set aside.

3. In a separate mixing bowl, whisk together the coconut oil, brown sugar, egg, vanilla, and salt until well blended. Pour the mixture into the dry ingredients and mix well with a rubber spatula. Fold in the apricots.

4. Using a 1-tablespoon measure, spoon the dough 2 inches apart onto the pre-pared baking sheets. Bake in the center of the oven for 10 to 12 minutes, or until cookies are lightly browned. Remove from the oven and set on racks to cool.

Ann's Tips

If you can't find whole-wheat pastry flour, mix a quarter cup whole-wheat flour with a quarter cup unbleached all-purpose flour.

Brown, unsulfured dried apricots won't win any beauty contests, but they are always the best, most natural choice. And besides, in a cookie like this, looks don't matter, just taste.

Lemon Yogurt Cake

HEALTH CONSIDERATIONS: IN TREATMENT; FATIGUE; EASY TO SWALLOW; NAUSEA; BLAND DIET; HIGH FIBER; HIGH CALORIE; NEUTROPENIC DIET

FOOD PREFERENCE: VEGETARIAN

Meal: Dessert, Snack

Main Ingredients: Yogurt, Whole-wheat flour

Prep Time: 30 minutes

Cook Time: 50 minutes

SERVES 8 TO 10

This delicious loaf cake is a breeze to make. I first ate it in Paris, where my friend Nuccia, who was no cook, would throw this together when people came over. It became known among her friends as the "impossible to ruin" cake. And it certainly is. The sweet-and-sour taste of the tart lemon glaze makes it a great choice for taste buds that are out of whack, and for those who simply enjoy the aroma of lemons baking and their excellent flavor.

1¼ cups whole-wheat pastry flour

2 teaspoons baking powder

½ teaspoon kosher salt

2 teaspoons grated lemon zest (from 1 small lemon)

1 cup whole-milk plain yogurt

1 cup plus 1 tablespoon organic granulated sugar, divided

3 extra-large eggs

½ teaspoon vanilla extract

½ cup extra-virgin olive oil

⅓ cup freshly squeezed lemon juice

1. Preheat the oven to 350°F. Grease and flour an 8½ x 4¼ x 2½-inch loaf pan. Line the bottom with parchment paper and set aside.

2. Sift together the flour, baking powder, and salt into a medium bowl. Stir in the lemon zest. Set aside.

3. In a separate large bowl, whisk together the yogurt, 1 cup of the sugar, the eggs, and vanilla. When blended, slowly whisk the dry ingredients into the wet ingredients until a batter forms.

4. Pour the batter into the prepared pan and bake for about 50 minutes, or until a toothpick inserted in the center of the loaf comes out clean. Transfer to a cool-

ing rack and let the cake cool in the pan for 10 minutes before turning it out onto the rack and removing the parchment paper.

5. Meanwhile, make the glaze: In a small pan, stir the remaining 1 tablespoon sugar with the lemon juice. Heat over medium heat until the sugar dissolves and the mixture is clear. While the cake is still warm (see Ann's Tips, below), set the cooling rack and cake over a sheet pan. Gradually spoon the lemon glaze over the cake until there is none left, allowing it to soak into the cake between spoonfuls. The sheet pan will catch any drips. Let cool. Serve in thick slices.

Ann's Tips

Prick the top of the warm cake with a toothpick. This will allow the glaze to sink more easily into the cake as you spoon it on.

This cake is very soft, but if your mouth is sore, maybe skip the lemon glaze.

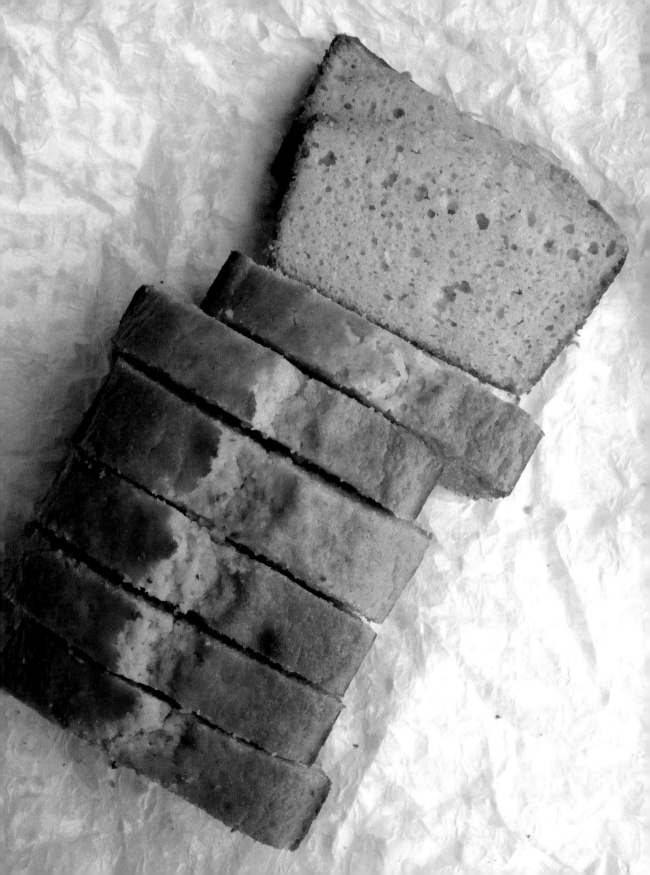

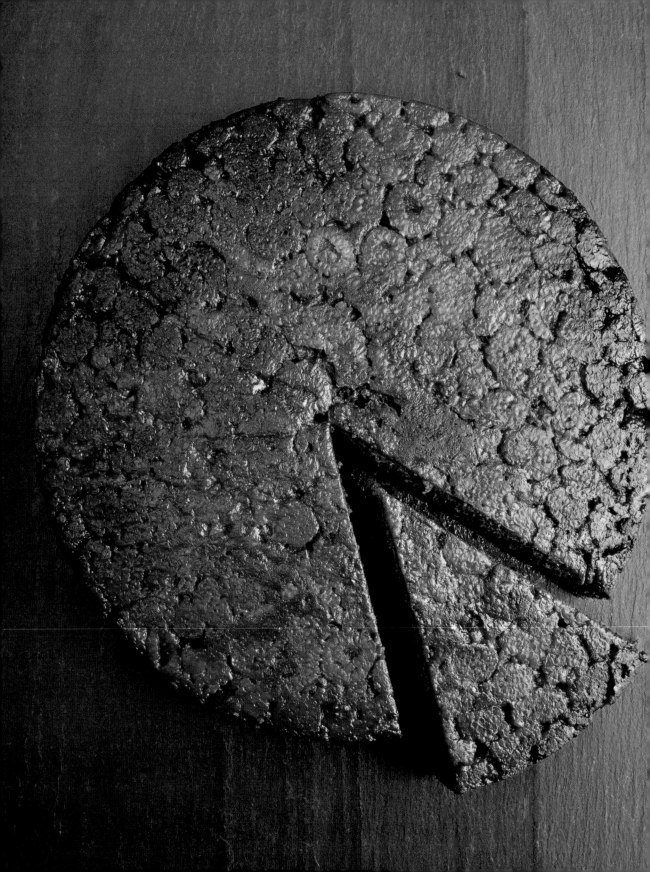

Chocolate-Raspberry Upside-Down Cake

Meal: Dessert

Main Ingredients:
Chocolate, Butter, Raspberries

Prep Time: 30 minutes

Bake Time: 35 to 40 minutes

SERVES 6 TO 8

HEALTH CONSIDERATIONS: IN TREATMENT; FATIGUE; HIGH FIBER; HIGH CALORIE; NEUTROPENIC DIET

FOOD PREFERENCE: VEGETARIAN

This is the perfect cake to make if you want a very special, very easy, very chocolaty treat. Chocolate goes well with many things but the combination with raspberries is one of my favorites. This dark, rich, almost fudgy upside-down cake is as straightforward to make as it is heavenly to eat. The cake is an all-in-one-bowl, the raspberries are frozen (so no prep there), and the parchment paper ensures that there will be no sticking as you turn the cake out.

10 tablespoons unsalted butter, melted

1½ cups frozen raspberries

1 cup plus 3 tablespoons granulated cane sugar, divided

¾ cup plus 2 tablespoons unsweetened cocoa powder

1 teaspoon vanilla extract

½ teaspoon sea salt

2 large eggs, at room temperature

½ cup whole-wheat pastry flour or unbleached all-purpose flour

1. Preheat the oven to 375°F. Grease an 8-inch cake pan with butter and line the bottom with parchment paper.
2. Toss the raspberries with 3 tablespoons of the sugar. Spread the raspberries in a single layer in the prepared pan. Set aside.
3. Beat the butter, the remaining 1 cup of sugar, the cocoa, vanilla, and salt in a medium bowl until the cocoa has been absorbed.

4. Add the eggs one at a time, stirring vigorously after each one. When the batter looks thick, shiny, and well blended, sift in the flour. Beat the batter vigorously for 30 seconds with a wooden spoon or a rubber spatula. The batter will be very thick. Spread evenly over the raspberries to about half an inch from the edge of the pan.

5. Bake 35 to 40 minutes, or until a toothpick plunged into the center emerges slightly moist. Let cool completely or for 1 hour before turning out onto a plate. Remove parchment and enjoy!

Ann's Tips

· ⌘ ·

You can use either natural or Dutch-processed unsweetened dark cocoa powder for this cake, but whatever you do, don't try to make this with powdered drinking chocolate. In general, I think Dutch-processed has the best flavor, but always check your recipe. As a rule of thumb, recipes that call for baking soda use natural cocoa powder, and those with baking powder use Dutch-processed cocoa. This is because "natural" cocoa powder is more acidic and gets balanced out by the baking soda.

This cake is very rich, so go easy. Although it's tempting, don't overindulge.

Orangey Tofu Chocolate Pudding

Meal: Snack, Dessert

Main Ingredient: Tofu

Prep Time: 10 minutes

Cook Time: 15 minutes, plus 30 to 40 minutes for chilling

SERVES 6 TO 8

HEALTH CONSIDERATIONS: IN TREATMENT; FATIGUE; EASY TO SWALLOW; BLAND DIET; LOW FIBER; GLUTEN-FREE; NEUTROPENIC DIET

FOOD PREFERENCE: DAIRY-FREE; VEGAN; VEGETARIAN

Chocolate and orange make a perfect marriage. This great, dairy-free pudding is always a huge hit when we make it in our classes. Not only is it simple to put together, it can safely be served to tofu haters; I swear they will never realize they're eating it.

8 ounces high-quality bittersweet or semisweet baking chocolate

¾ cup organic granulated cane sugar

¾ cup water

2 teaspoons grated orange zest

¾ pound silken tofu

Candied orange peel or julienned orange zest, for decoration (optional)

1. Bring 2 to 3 inches of water to a simmer in a large saucepan set over medium heat.
2. Break the chocolate into pieces and place it in a heatproof bowl over the saucepan, making sure the bowl does not touch the water. Stir the chocolate often until completely melted, 10 to 12 minutes.
3. Meanwhile, combine the sugar, water, and orange zest in a small saucepan and bring to a boil. Cook, stirring occasionally, until the sugar is dissolved. Cool slightly.
4. Place sugar mixture, melted chocolate, and tofu into the blender and puree until completely smooth, stopping the machine to scrape down its sides if necessary. Transfer the pudding to a large bowl and chill for at least 30 minutes. Garnish with candied orange peel, if using, just before serving.

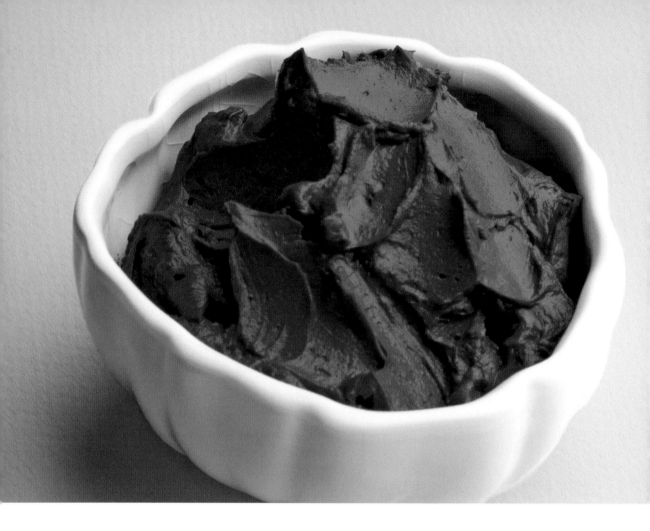

Ann's Tips

· ⚜ ·

Don't skimp on the chocolate. Use the very best dark bittersweet or semisweet baking chocolate you can find, such as Callebaut or Valrhona. It's well worth it. If speed is of the essence, buy Ghirardelli bittersweet chocolate chips for faster melting.

This dessert is very rich. If you want to keep tabs on portion size, instead of serving this family style, divide the pudding among eight 4-ounce ramekins before chilling.

Apple and Raspberry Coconut Crumble

Meal: Dessert

Main Ingredients:
Apples, Frozen raspberries, Coconut

Prep Time: 30 minutes, plus 30 minutes for freezing

Bake Time: 35 minutes

SERVES 6

HEALTH CONSIDERATIONS: IN TREATMENT; NAUSEA; NEUTROPENIC DIET; BLAND DIET

FOOD PREFERENCE: DAIRY-FREE; VEGAN; VEGETARIAN

This ever-so-slightly naughty dessert is completely scrumptious and totally vegan. It's similar to a favorite English dessert served in the fall that combines blackberries with apples. But I think using a tartly pleasing frozen fruit like raspberries is an even better way to mix things up. Why? Because you can do it year-round, and in the late winter, just when you think you can't face another apple, this dessert makes them new again. Coconut oil is a great substitute for butter in baking, particularly for pastries and crumbles. Like butter, coconut oil hardens when cold to provide the wonderful shortness that makes these crusts so delicious.

Health Tip

Coconut oil, while high in saturated fat, is rich in lauric acid, a strong antibacterial agent. This recipe can easily be made using gluten-free oats and flour.

Use all-purpose flour if you are on a bland diet.

Coconut Crumble Topping

1 cup plus 3 tablespoons whole-wheat pastry flour

⅓ cup unsweetened desiccated shredded coconut

⅓ cup rolled oats

½ cup organic granulated sugar (see Ann's Tips, page 257)

(continued)

¾ teaspoon ground ginger (optional)

¾ teaspoon sea salt, or to taste

½ cup coconut oil, melted (see Ann's Tips, next page)

Filling

2 to 3 Golden Delicious or Gala apples (about 1½ pounds), peeled, cored, and thickly sliced (see Ann's Tips, next page)

1 cup frozen raspberries

1 tablespoon lemon juice

2 tablespoons organic granulated sugar, or to taste

1. Line a small baking sheet with parchment paper and set aside.

2. Make the topping: In a large bowl, stir together 1 cup plus 2 tablespoons of the flour, and the coconut, oats, sugar, ginger, and salt with a fork until well blended. Make a well in the center and pour in the coconut oil. Start to mix together with the fork until you have a lumpy mixture. Dust with the remaining 1 tablespoon of flour and gently rub the ingredients together with your fingertips just until the crumble looks like chunky bread crumbs. Don't overmix. Spread onto a prepared baking sheet, cover with plastic wrap, and freeze for at least 1 hour, or until you are ready to bake. Chilling will make the crumble crisper. (You can make this ahead of time.)

3. When you are ready to bake the crumble, preheat the oven to 375°F. Grease a 1.5-quart (11 x 7 x 2-inch) baking dish and set aside.

4. Prepare the filling: In a large bowl, toss the apples and raspberries together. Add lemon juice and toss, then add sugar and mix until the fruit is coated. The raspberries will start to thaw, but this is okay. Spoon the fruit into the prepared baking dish in an even layer.

5. Take the crumble topping from the freezer and quickly break it up with your fingers or a fork. Sprinkle it over the fruit. Bake for 30 to 35 minutes, or until lightly browned and crisp, and the fruit is juicy and bubbling under the edges of the topping. Allow to sit for 10 minutes. Serve warm or at room temperature.

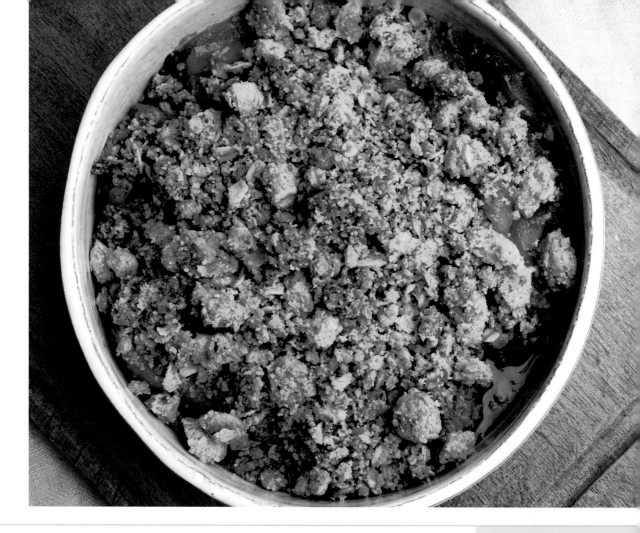

Most supermarket apples weigh between 8 and 9 ounces each. If you buy apples at the greenmarket, they will possibly be smaller and you may need to use more than 3 apples.

We've purposely used sweet apples for this dish to cut down on the need to add sugar. If you prefer tarter apples such as Granny Smiths or Braeburns, however, you may need to add a little more sugar to the filling.

To melt coconut oil, simply stand the jar in a bowl of hot water.

You can freeze and bag the crumble topping and keep it ready to make quick desserts.

Ann's
Tips

· ⚛ ·

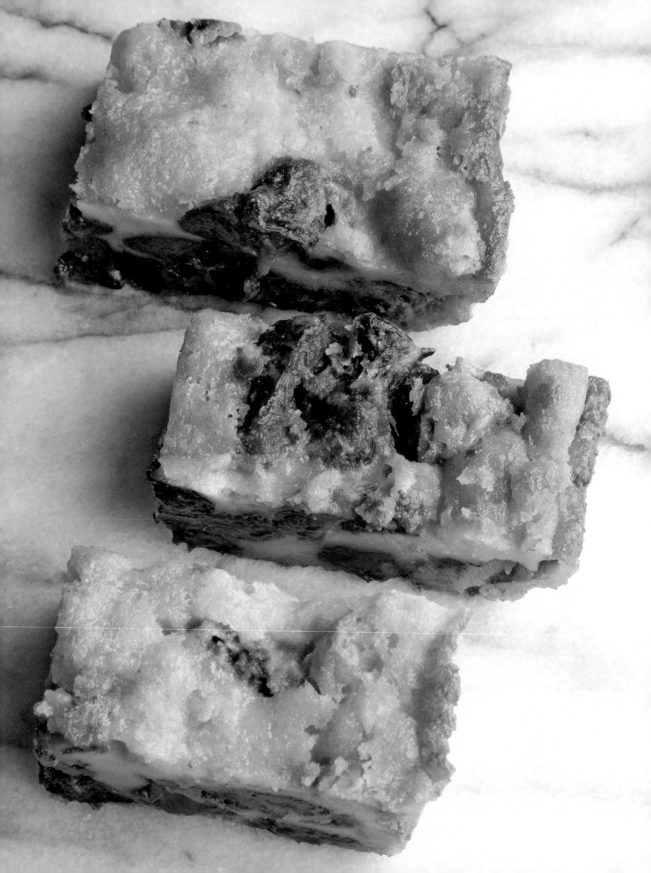

Prune Clafoutis

HEALTH CONSIDERATIONS: IN TREATMENT; EASY TO SWALLOW; NAUSEA; HIGH FIBER; NEUTROPENIC DIET

FOOD PREFERENCE: VEGETARIAN

Meal: Dessert

Main Ingredients: Prunes, Eggs, Butter

Prep Time: 30 minutes

Cook Time: 40 minutes

SERVES 6

Clafoutis is a simple, rustic dessert that over the centuries has become a French classic. It originated in the Limousin region of central France and is basically a thick, rich pancake made with stone fruit baked in. It has the added bonus of being easy to put together. This recipe is a version that my friend Christine makes, which I ate at her house in the Auvergne. I make it with prunes, which I adore. They are so good for us that I always have them in my pantry. Usually humble and toiling away at keeping us regular, prunes are the stars of this rich-tasting dessert. Fiber never tasted so good.

Health Tip

If you are on a neutropenic diet, check with your doctor to ensure it's safe for you to consume probiotics during treatment before eating this with yogurt.

7 tablespoons unsalted butter, divided

⅔ cup whole-wheat pastry flour or unbleached all-purpose flour

⅔ cup organic cane sugar

⅓ cup cornstarch

½ teaspoon fine sea salt

6 large eggs, lightly beaten

1 cup plus 2 tablespoons milk

1 teaspoon lemon zest

1 tablespoon maple syrup

2 cups hot water

½ pound pitted prunes (see Ann's Tips, next page)

Plain Greek yogurt or crème fraîche, for serving (optional)

1. In a small saucepan melt 6 tablespoons of the butter over low heat until it foams. Set aside.
2. Sift the flour, sugar, and cornstarch together into a large mixing bowl. Stir in the salt. Make a well in the center of the flour mixture. Using a handheld mixer, gradually beat in the eggs. Slowly beat in the milk and add the melted butter. Beat until you have a smooth batter. Cover and leave in the fridge to chill while you prepare the prunes.
3. In a 2-quart saucepan, mix the lemon zest, maple syrup, and hot water. Add the prunes and bring to a boil. Cover, remove from the heat, and leave the prunes to soak for 30 minutes. Drain and quarter the prunes.
4. Preheat the oven to 350°F. Butter a 2-quart (13 x 9 x 2-inch) baking dish with 1 teaspoon of the butter and set it on a baking sheet for easier handling. Spread the prunes evenly in the dish and dot with the remaining butter. Pour the batter over the prunes and bake in the oven on a middle rack for 40 minutes, or until the clafoutis is golden and puffy and a toothpick inserted in the center comes out clean.
5. Serve warm or at room temperature with a dollop of thick Greek yogurt (see Health Tip, previous page) or some crème fraîche. If you eat it cold, dust it with a little confectioners' sugar before serving.

Ann's Tips

· ✲ ·

With prunes, bigger isn't better. Avoid the large California prunes, which are actually dried round black plums and have quite a different flavor. For best results, use the prunes that come from drying the small oblong Italian plums. If you can find the French Pruneaux d'Agen variety, use them; they are totally delicious.

Apples Baked with Dates and Walnuts

Meal: Dessert

Main Ingredient: Apples

Prep Time: 20 minutes

Cook Time: 40 to 45 minutes

SERVES 4

HEALTH CONSIDERATIONS: BLAND DIET; GLUTEN-FREE; IN TREATMENT; EASY TO SWALLOW (SEE HEALTH TIP, BELOW); NAUSEA; FATIGUE; NEUTROPENIC DIET

FOOD PREFERENCE: VEGETARIAN; NUTS

This simple and simply delicious dessert is a great way to get fruit into your diet no matter where you are in treatment. Golden Russet and Braeburn apples are on the tart side and get fluffy when cooked, both perfect attributes for a baking apple. Their tartness goes well with sweet, naturally sugary dates, and their fluffiness makes for easy eating. This recipe is for regular supermarket-size apples, which are about 8 ounces each—you may need less filling for smaller greenmarket apples.

4 Golden Russet or Braeburn apples, washed and cored

4 dates, pitted and halved, or more to taste

½ cup roughly chopped walnuts

2 tablespoons maple syrup

2 teaspoons unsalted butter (optional)

1 teaspoon organic granulated sugar (see Ann's Tips, next page)

1 tablespoon water (optional)

Greek yogurt, for serving (optional)

Health Tip

If the walnuts are too rough for a sore mouth or throat or you are allergic to them, leave them out. If you are on a neutropenic diet, check with your doctor to ensure it's safe for you to consume probiotics during treatment before eating this with yogurt.

1. Preheat the oven to 400°F.
2. Slit the skin of the apples around their middles, but don't cut deep into the flesh. Set the apples in a baking dish just big enough to hold them.
3. Stuff the center of each apple with a half date, some walnuts, another half date, and top with a few more walnuts. Set aside any walnuts that are left over. Drizzle the maple syrup over the apples, making sure that some goes into the stuffed

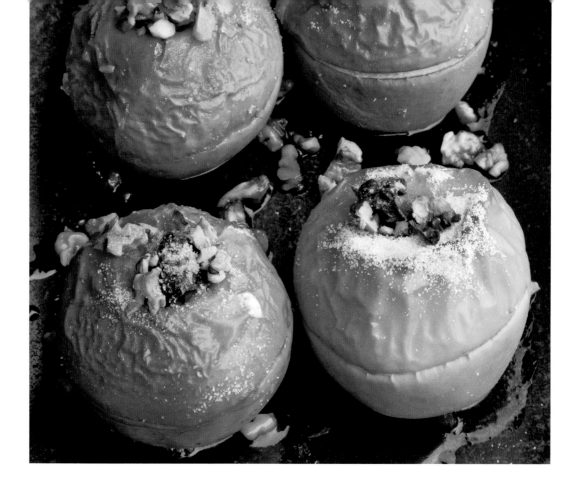

centers. Dot the top of the filling with butter, if using, and sprinkle with the sugar. Add the water to the bottom of the dish, if using.

4. Bake on the center rack of the oven for 20 minutes. Sprinkle the apples with the remaining walnuts and return to the oven to bake for 20 to 25 minutes more, or until the apples have swelled and opened the slit in the skin around their middles and the tops are browned. Serve warm with Greek yogurt.

Ann's
Tips

· ·

If you'd rather not use added sweeteners, use a sweeter variety of apple such as Gala or Golden Delicious.

Poached-Pear Bread Pudding

HEALTH CONSIDERATIONS: IN TREATMENT; EASY TO SWALLOW; NAUSEA;
BLAND DIET; LOW FIBER; NEUTROPENIC DIET; HEALTHY SURVIVORSHIP

FOOD PREFERENCE: VEGETARIAN

Meal: Dessert

Main Ingredients: Bread, Eggs, Milk, Pears

Prep Time: 20 minutes

Cook Time: 45 minutes

SERVES 6

I've always loved bread puddings. They are so easy to eat, especially when you don't feel great. You can use any kind of bread, but for those on a bland or low-fiber diet, a simple white bread is perfect for making this soothing dessert. Although not overly sweet, the layers of gingered poached pears add a cool, spicy sweetness to this simple pudding. You can also use canned pears if you aren't up to making the microwave ones, and add the candied ginger. It will make them sing.

4 halves Microwave Gingered Pears (page 92), drained, or canned pears, drained (see Ann's Tips, next page)

2 cups whole or 2% milk

3 eggs, lightly beaten

3 tablespoons organic granulated cane sugar, or to taste, divided

Zest of 1 small lemon

½ teaspoon grated nutmeg

¼ teaspoon vanilla extract (optional)

2 tablespoons unsalted butter, or to taste, at room temperature

6 (8 x ½-inch-thick) slices unbleached white bread, sourdough, or Pullman, crusts removed (see Ann's Tips, next page)

6 to 8 pieces candied ginger, roughly chopped into small pieces, divided (optional)

1. Preheat the oven to 350°F. Grease a nonreactive 1-quart oval baking dish or 9 x 6 x 2-inch loaf pan. Set aside. Bring a kettle of water to a boil.
2. Slice the drained pears lengthwise into ¼-inch-thick slices. Set aside.
3. In a medium bowl, whisk the milk into the beaten eggs a little at a time until it is all used up. Add 2 tablespoons of the sugar. Whisk until the sugar is dissolved. Stir in the lemon zest, nutmeg, and vanilla, if using.

4. Lightly butter all the bread slices and cut across into triangles—it will help you fit them all in the baking dish. Line the dish with a single layer of bread, buttered-side up. Sprinkle with one-third of the ginger, if using, then layer on roughly one-third of the pears. Repeat, ending with a layer of bread. Pour the egg mixture over the bread. It should almost cover the top slice without submerging it. Sprinkle the top with the remaining 1 tablespoon sugar and dot with the remaining butter.

5. Set the baking dish into another larger ovenproof dish and put into the oven. Carefully fill the ovenproof dish with the reserved hot water so that it comes two-thirds of the way up the sides of the pudding dish. Bake for 45 to 50 minutes, or until set and a toothpick inserted in the center comes out clean. Serve in thick slices, warm or at room temperature.

Ann's Tips

· ✦ ·

If you make the microwaved pears, reserve the juice—it is gingery and tasty. Spoon over the cooked bread pudding or add it to smoothies.

Some notes about the amounts of bread needed:

- Before buttering the slices, take 6 slices and see how well they fit into your chosen dish, then add more if needed. If you use a baguette, start with twelve ½-inch-thick slices.
- If your bread is presliced, it may be thinner than the recipe asks for, and you will need to use more, possibly even double the number of slices. If this is the case, alternate the candied ginger and the sliced pears between the layers of bread, ending with a layer of bread as per the recipe directions.

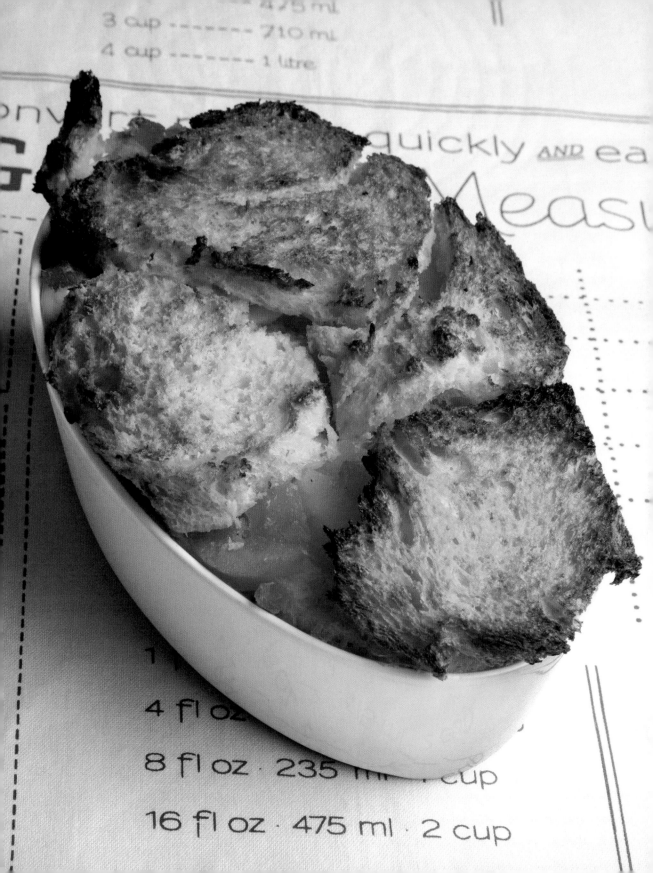

Maple-Poached Apples

Meal: Breakfast; Dessert

Main Ingredient: Apples

Prep Time: 20 minutes

Cook Time: 20 minutes

SERVES 4

HEALTH CONSIDERATIONS: IN TREATMENT; FATIGUE; NAUSEA; BLAND DIET; LOW FIBER; GLUTEN-FREE; NEUTROPENIC DIET; HEALTHY SURVIVORSHIP; EASY TO SWALLOW

FOOD PREFERENCE: DAIRY-FREE; VEGAN; VEGETARIAN

These are my version of applesauce. Don't worry about the limited amount of liquid, the apples have plenty of their own juice to give up. What is important is to have a tight-fitting lid so that they can steam in their own juices. The apples we've used here are tart-sweet and keep their shape, as that's how I like them—but by all means, break them up if you prefer it. If you have a sweet tooth, you don't need to add more sugar, just use a sweeter apple such as Golden Delicious or Honeycrisp.

5 medium tart-sweet apples, such as Braeburn, Pink Lady, or Golden Russets if you can find them

2 tablespoons maple syrup

2 to 3 tablespoons water

3 whole cloves

Whole milk or 2% plain Greek yogurt, for serving (optional)

1. Peel, core, and cut each apple into 8 wedges. Place the wedges into a heavy pot with a lid (see Ann's Tips, next page). Add the maple syrup and the water and tuck in the cloves.
2. Bring the liquid to a boil over high heat. Reduce the heat to medium-low and cook, covered, until the apples are soft but not falling apart, about 30 minutes. Turn off the heat, keeping the pot covered, and allow the apples to cool. They will continue cooking as the pot cools down. Serve as is or with a dollop of plain Greek yogurt.

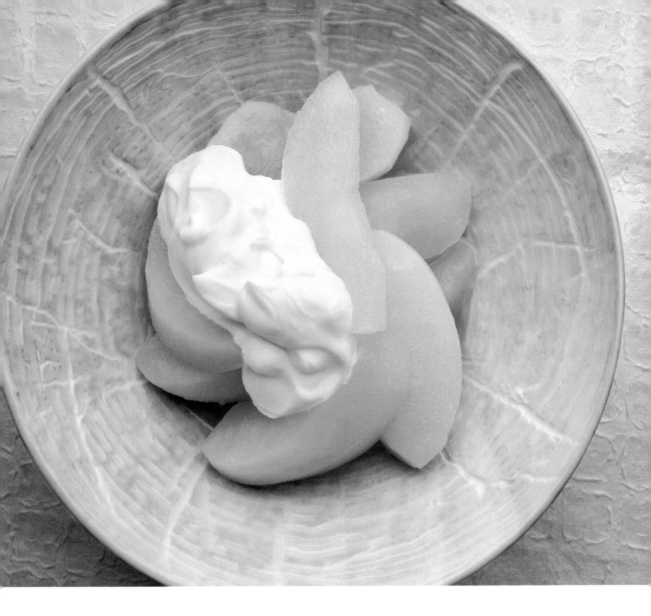

If your lid doesn't fit too well, loosely cover the top of the pot with either foil or a dish towel and put the lid on. This will seal it nicely.

Ann's Tips

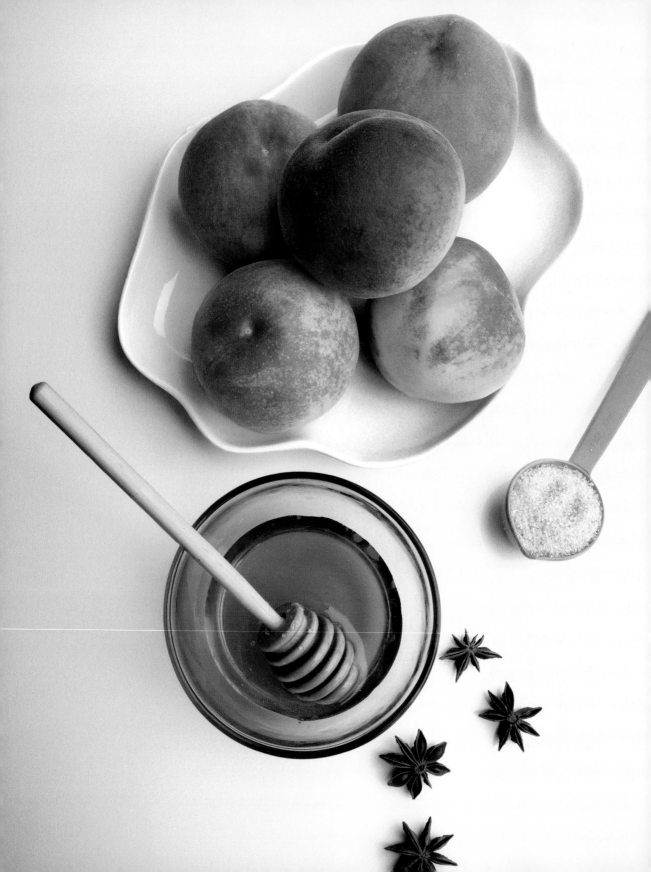

Peaches Poached in Honey

HEALTH CONSIDERATIONS: IN TREATMENT; FATIGUE; EASY TO SWALLOW; NAUSEA; BLAND DIET; LOW FIBER; GLUTEN-FREE; NEUTROPENIC DIET

FOOD PREFERENCE: DAIRY-FREE; VEGETARIAN

Meal: Dessert

Main Ingredient: Peaches

Prep Time: 30 minutes

Cook Time: 25 minutes

SERVES 6

I just love fresh, ripe peaches, and was devastated when during treatment I was told I could eat canned fruit, but not fresh. The idea of eating these sugar-laden versions of the real thing just didn't sit well with me. Then I thought about how I used to poach peaches in wine and figured I could use the method, minus the alcohol, to get around the ban. This easy summer dessert is what I came up with. Star anise gives a lovely flavor to the light poaching syrup, but if you can't find any, the honey makes the peaches quite delicious on their own. Served chilled for a wonderfully refreshing treat on a hot day, and if you are on a neutropenic diet, as I was, you'll finally have a tasty way to eat a fruit that would otherwise be off the menu without having to resort to canned fruit.

6 to 8 ripe yellow or white peaches

2 tablespoons honey, or to taste (see Ann's Tips, next page)

1 tablespoon sugar (optional)

1½ cups cold water

1 piece star anise (see Ann's Tips, next page)

1. In a large sauté pan, bring to a simmer enough water to cover the peaches. Fill a bowl with ice water and set aside.
2. Put the peaches into the simmering water and blanch about 2 minutes, or until the skins start to look dull. Remove from the hot water with a slotted spoon, and plunge into the ice water.
3. Cut the peaches in half vertically through the stem ends and twist. The skins will come off very easily. Split the peaches open along the cut and remove the

pits. Place the peaches, cut-sides down, into a clean sauté pan or deep frying pan, preferably one with a lid.

4. When all the peaches have been skinned and halved, discard the ice water. Drizzle the peaches with honey and sprinkle with sugar, if using. Pour 1½ cups fresh water over them and add the star anise. Bring to a simmer over medium-high heat, then cover and reduce the heat to low. Simmer for 20 to 25 minutes, or until the peaches are just soft. Turn off the heat, keeping the pan covered, and leave the peaches to cool. When cool, remove the anise and chill the peaches and poaching syrup. Serve chilled, with syrup spooned over the peaches.

Ann's Tips

Slipping the skins off is easy to do when the peaches are ripe. If you make this recipe when peaches are out of season, you will probably be better off skipping step 2 and simply using a peeler on them.

The better the grade of honey you use, the better this will taste. I prefer clear orange blossom or other flowered honey for this dish.

If you can't find star anise, substitute either half a cinnamon stick or use no spice at all.

One of my favorite kitchen gadgets is the universal lid. These grooved stainless steel lids are designed to snugly fit a number of different-diameter pans. I have two, one to fit small pans 5 to 8 inches wide, and another for 9 to 12 inches. They will turn any frying pan into a fabulous poaching pan.

Honey-Roasted Plums

HEALTH CONSIDERATIONS: IN TREATMENT; EASY TO SWALLOW; NAUSEA; BLAND DIET (SEE HEALTH TIP, BELOW); GLUTEN-FREE; NEUTROPENIC DIET

FOOD PREFERENCE: DAIRY-FREE; VEGETARIAN; NUTS

Meal: Dessert

Main Ingredient: Plums

Prep Time: 15 minutes

Cook Time: 30 minutes

SERVES 6 TO 8

Roasting fruit is a great way to bring out their natural sweetness and make them safe to eat when you're in chemo. You'll find that even with the added sugar these plums are still pleasantly tart—they're the perfect treat when accompanied by creamy Greek yogurt. And they make great leftovers to eat for breakfast or anytime!

Health Tip

If you are on a bland diet, you may want to pass on both the almonds and the yogurt as a garnish. If you are on a neutropenic diet, you may need to avoid adding a dollop of probiotic yogurt. Ask your registered dietician or doctor.

---

3 tablespoons light brown or organic granulated cane sugar

6 ripe, round black or red plums, halved and pitted

1 tablespoon water (optional; see Ann's Tips, next page)

2 tablespoons honey

½ cup plain full-fat or 2% Greek yogurt (optional; see Health Tip, above)

¼ cup toasted sliced almonds

1. Preheat the oven to 400°F. Grease a baking dish large enough to hold the fruit tightly in a single layer. Depending on the size of your plums, a 1½-quart (10 x 8 x 1¾-inch) baking dish should do it. Set the baking dish aside.

2. Tip the sugar into a medium bowl. Add the plums, toss to coat, and allow them to sit for 10 minutes to macerate. Add 1 tablespoon of water, if using, to the greased dish. Transfer the plums to the dish in one layer. It doesn't matter if you

have to cram them in; they'll shrink as they cook in the oven. Drizzle the plums with the honey.

3. Roast on a middle rack in the oven until the sugar is bubbling and the plums are browned and syrupy-looking, 35 to 40 minutes. Let cool slightly. Serve with a dollop of Greek yogurt, if using, and sprinkled with toasted sliced almonds.

Ann's Tips

· ✻ ·

You can make this quick, yummy dessert with any type of plum. Keep in mind, though, that cooking times will depend on the type of plum you use, and you may need to add the water for the bigger varietals. Small black Italian plums will only need 20 to 25 minutes, and no water. Allow 2 per person instead of 1.

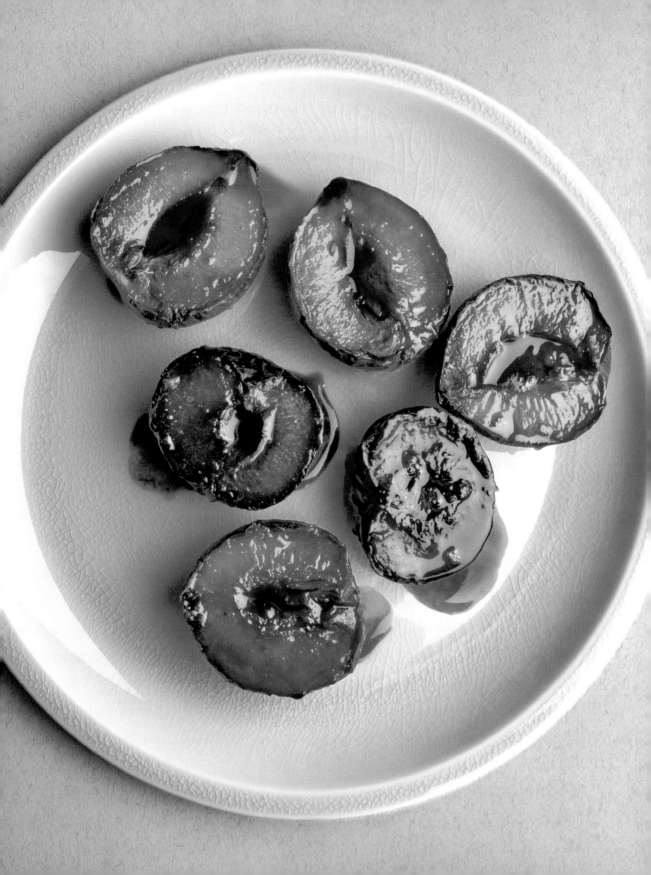

Raspberry Seltzer Cooler

Meal: Snack, Beverage

Main Ingredient: Frozen raspberries

Prep Time: 5 minutes

Cook Time: 0 minutes

SERVES 6

HEALTH CONSIDERATIONS: IN TREATMENT; FATIGUE; EASY TO SWALLOW; NAUSEA; BLAND DIET; LOW FIBER; GLUTEN-FREE; HEALTHY SURVIVORSHIP

FOOD PREFERENCE: DAIRY-FREE; VEGAN; VEGETARIAN

This is a wonderfully easy way to make a delectable cooler that's low calorie and uses real food as its ingredients. Once you're done, you can even reuse the berries in a smoothie. Coolers like this are also great if you are trying to cut down on soda. You don't need ice because the frozen berries pull double duty here. You can top up the pitcher with seltzer as you go.

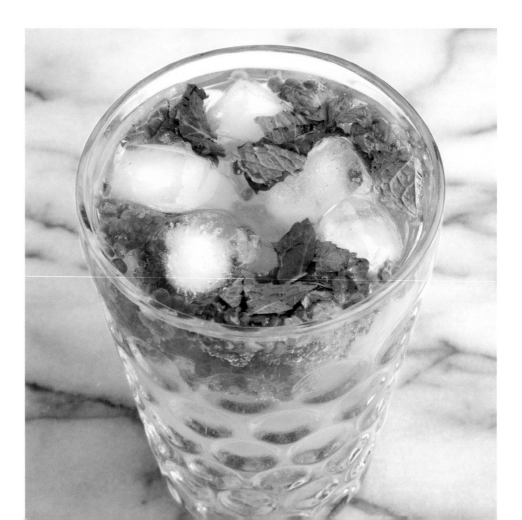

½ (16-ounce) bag frozen raspberries

3 to 4 sprigs mint, leaves stripped

1 (32-ounce) bottle plain, unflavored seltzer water

2 teaspoons agave nectar or honey, or to taste (optional; see Ann's Tips, below)

Ice (optional)

1. Place the frozen raspberries into a large pitcher. Crush the mint leaves in your hand to release their oils and add to the berries. Cover with the seltzer water and stir in the agave, if using. Let steep for 5 minutes. Serve with ice, if desired.

Ann's Tips

·✵·

If you are trying to rein in your sweet tooth, drinks are a great place to start, either with a refreshing fruity summer cooler like this, but especially with your daily coffee and tea. Ultra-sweet synthetic sweeteners may not add calories but they do keep your sweet tooth alive and craving more sweets. Cut them out and use real sugars in your drinks instead, but over 3 or 4 weeks, gradually cut down on the amount you add, half a teaspoon at a time, until you arrive at zero. Agave nectar and honey dissolve well in liquids but, spoon for spoon, are twice as sweet, so bear that in mind if you use these. Once you lose your added sugar habit, you'll find you no longer enjoy nor crave the taste of overly sweet drinks and foods. And you won't be automatically adding all those empty calories to your daily diet, either.

Scrumptious

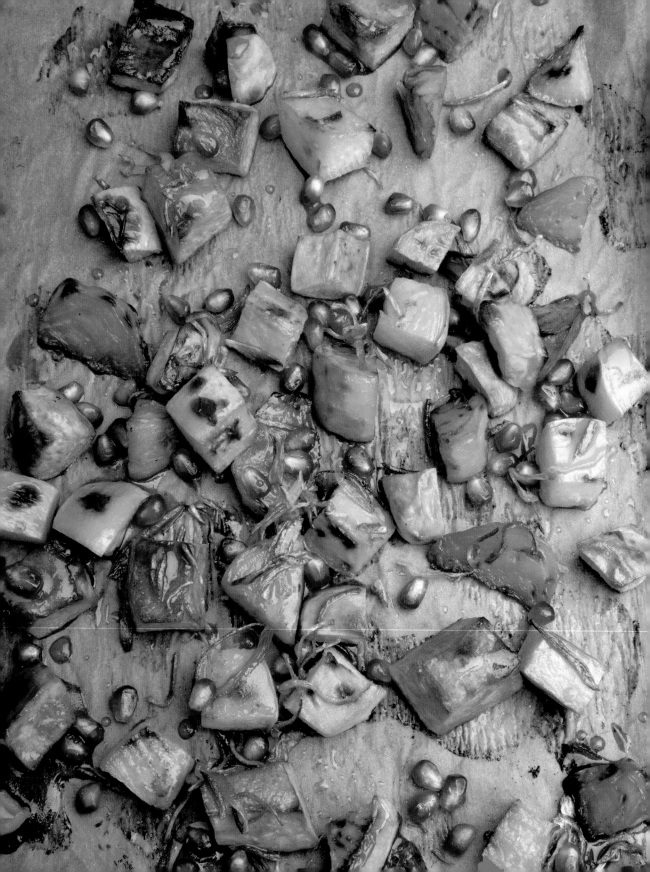

For me, this describes the truly wonderful moment that I had looked forward to throughout my entire treatment: its end. My hair grew back, my taste buds returned to normal, and all food started to taste good again. I was able to indulge once more in all the wonderful, delicious, fresh foods that I wasn't able to risk eating when I was in treatment. I welcomed back onto my plate deliciously crunchy fresh raw salads, succulent fresh fruits and berries, briny shrimp and shellfish, even Brie and blue cheese. In my kitchen, I said good-bye to the necessity of dealing with my side effects. I started to concentrate on cooking great-tasting food that would keep me healthy. Scrumptious food.

Eating healthily is all about scrumptiousness, otherwise there's no point. Healthy food is too often synonymous with dullness and lack of flavor, not to mention a ton of restrictions. Cancer treatment comes with its own necessarily severe dietary restraints, and I for one couldn't wait to throw them off. Scrumptiousness explores using juicy fruits, crunchy whole grains, leafy greens, farm-raised chicken and eggs, and wild-caught seafood . . . I could go on. Basically it means using ingredients as good as you can afford, simply and deliciously cooked. This is healthy food.

These recipes are a paean to the freedom I felt once my energy was back and I could return to the kitchen to play. I remember the day that I presented my husband, Joe, with a steaming dish of mussels cooked in white wine, the kind of dish that we had both missed so much when I was ill. It was scrumptious. I knew then that my inner cook was back. Yours will show up again, too.

Healthy food that nourishes and protects doesn't have to be boring, but it must be scrumptious. Enjoy!

Warm Grilled Shrimp and Leek Salad

Meal: Main

Main Ingredients: Shrimp, Leeks, Arugula

Prep Time: 10 minutes

Cook Time: 10 minutes

SERVES 2 TO 4

HEALTH CONSIDERATIONS: GLUTEN-FREE; IN TREATMENT; HIGH FIBER; HEALTHY SURVIVORSHIP; FATIGUE

FOOD PREFERENCE: DAIRY-FREE

I love shrimp. It's quick cooking, low in calories, high in protein and vitamin B_{12}, and even has omega-3s. And along with all that good stuff, it tastes terrific. I also love leeks. Grilling is an easy, flavorful way to cook leeks that brings out all their sweetness. Add lemony shrimp to the grill with them, and toss both together in a simple vinaigrette with some spicy cruciferous arugula. What you'll have is a nutrient-packed meal fit for a gourmet.

Health Tip

Shrimp is back on the American Heart Association's heart-healthy food list. Worries about its cholesterol are now past. But try to buy shrimp from US farms, which are closely regulated.

Juice of ½ lemon

3 tablespoons plus 2 teaspoons extra-virgin olive oil, divided

½ pound large shrimp, peeled and deveined

2 large leeks, white parts only, roughly shredded and rinsed (see Ann's Tips, next page)

1 tablespoon cider vinegar

Sea salt, to taste

3 cups arugula, washed

1. In a medium bowl, mix the lemon juice with 2 teaspoons of the oil. Add the shrimp and stir to coat with the marinade. Set aside in a cool place while you prep and cook the leeks.

2. Heat a cast-iron grill over medium-high heat and brush with some of the remaining oil. Lay the shredded leeks on the hot grill. Cook, turning from time to time, until they have softened and have some brown spots, about 8 minutes. If you don't have a cast-iron grill pan, check out Ann's Tips, below.

3. While the leeks are grilling, whisk the cider vinegar, a generous pinch of salt, and the remaining oil together in a salad bowl. Set aside.

4. When the leeks are ready, push them to one side of the grill, leaving the hot center open. Lay the shrimp on the grill in one layer. Brush with any remaining marinade and sprinkle with a little salt. Cook until they start to turn pink underneath, about 2 minutes, then turn and cook the other side until just pink. Do not overcook or they'll be tough.

5. Quickly mix the shrimp with the leeks on the grill, then transfer everything to the salad bowl with the dressing and toss together. Add the arugula on top and toss again quickly (the arugula will wilt). Serve immediately.

Ann's Tips

· 𝍫 ·

To shred leeks, cut them in half across and then roughly shred them down their length. I find this easiest to do by halving then quartering them, and then halving the quarters again. Wash well then pat dry on paper towels. Set aside.

If you don't have a cast-iron grill pan, preheat a heavy nonstick pan, toss the leeks in 1 to 2 teaspoons of olive oil, and spread them out on the hot pan. Cook until they start to soften and brown around the edges. Turn them with a spatula, and continue with step 4.

For information on sustainable fish choices, go to the Monterey Bay Aquarium's Seafood Watch website, seafoodwatch.org.

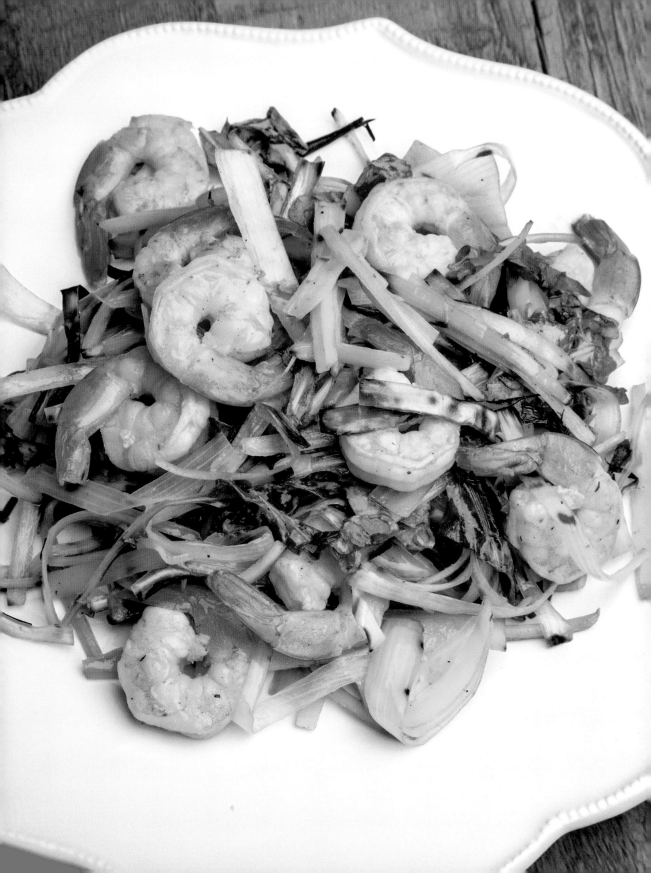

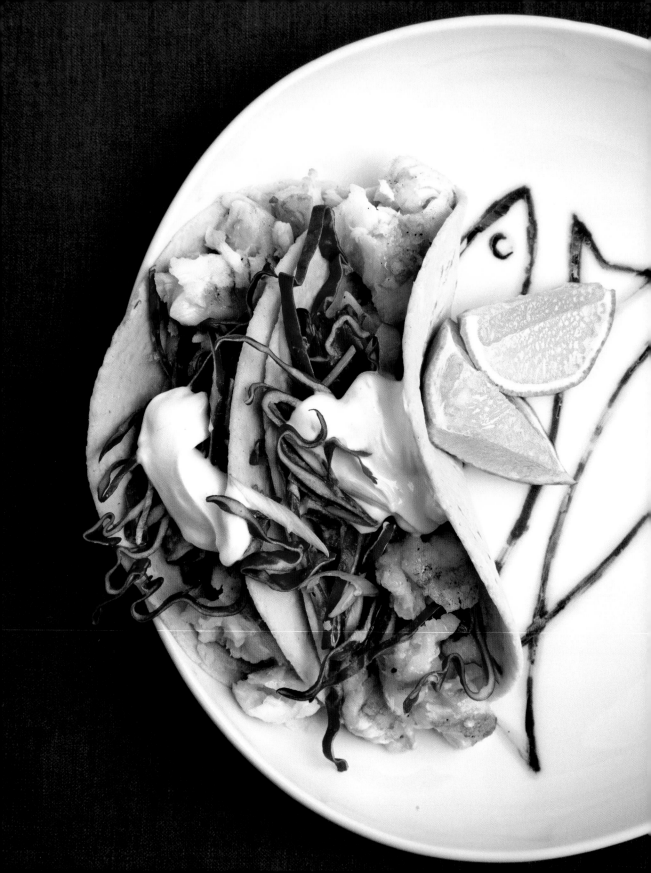

Fish Tacos with Red Cabbage Slaw

HEALTH CONSIDERATIONS: IN TREATMENT; FATIGUE; HIGH FIBER; GLUTEN-FREE; HEALTHY SURVIVORSHIP

FOOD PREFERENCE: NONE

Fish tacos are great, and this recipe is one of the best. It looks more complicated to make than it is—basically, it's just a piece of marinated fish, broiled then popped into a soft tortilla with a simple red cabbage slaw. Just follow the directions and all will be perfectly easy. If you want to get a head start, the slaw in these tacos can be made ahead of time. Red cabbage can sometimes be bought precut—a great way to simplify prep, so buy it if you see it. Unlike salads of soft lettuce greens, cabbage salads actually improve with keeping. The vinaigrette dressing "cooks" and softens the leaves. Keep it in the fridge to have something nutritious to snack on for a couple of days, if it lasts that long without being eaten.

Meal: Main
Main Ingredients: Fish; Red cabbage
Prep Time: 30 minutes, plus 20 minutes for marinating
Cook Time: 15 minutes
SERVES 4 TO 6

Marinade

2 tablespoons grapeseed or canola oil

Juice of 1 medium lime

1 small jalapeño, minced

¼ cup chopped cilantro

¾ pound mild flaky white-flesh fish (cod, haddock, hake)

Red Cabbage Slaw with Honey-Mustard Vinaigrette

2 tablespoons cider vinegar

½ teaspoon Dijon mustard

1 teaspoon honey

3 tablespoons extra-virgin olive oil

Sea salt and freshly ground black pepper, to taste

(continued)

½ small red onion, sliced

3 scallions, white and green parts, sliced

¼ cup chopped cilantro

½ head medium red cabbage, shredded (about 2 cups)

4 (6-inch) corn tortillas

Greek yogurt, to taste

Lime wedges

1. Make the marinade: In a medium bowl, whisk together the oil, lime juice, jalapeño, and cilantro. Place the fish in the dish, and turn to coat. Let marinate for 15 to 20 minutes.
2. Meanwhile, make the slaw: In a bowl, whisk together the vinegar, mustard, honey, oil, and salt and pepper to taste. Add the onion, scallions, cilantro, and red cabbage. Toss well until all the cabbage is coated with dressing. Set aside while you cook the fish.
3. Heat the grill or broiler to medium-high. Remove the fish from the marinade and place on the grill. Cook for 3 minutes, then turn and cook for another minute or so, or until the fish is cooked through. Let rest for 5 minutes, then with a fork flake the fish into bite-size pieces.
4. Place the tortillas on the grill for 20 seconds, then divide the fish among the tortillas and top with the slaw and a dollop of Greek yogurt. Serve with lime wedges.

Ann's Tips
· ❋ ·

Red cabbage is often slow-cooked, but this slaw offers a great way to enjoy it on the fly. All cabbages are rich in glucosinolates, a group of phytonutrients that studies show could aid in protecting from cancer. Rather than focusing on one particular kind of cabbage, it seems we should eat as many different types as possible to get the most benefit. So the next time you make slaw, go red.

Chiles Rellenos

HEALTH CONSIDERATIONS: IN TREATMENT; GLUTEN-FREE; NEUTROPENIC DIET

FOOD PREFERENCE: VEGETARIAN

This tasty, baked version of the fried Tex-Mex classic mixes cheese with quinoa for a lower fat content, but you could use any cooked grain for this. Chiles rellenos is notoriously hard to make at home, but relatively speaking, this is one of the easiest ways to achieve a seriously satisfying result. Stuffing the peppers is admittedly a little fiddly, but once you get going, it's easy and well worth the effort to have something so tasty. The recipe is also easy to divide if you want to make only one or two of these tasty peppers. Serve with a crisp green salad and our spicy Quick Tomato Sauce (page 27) or in the morning with eggs. It's also great topped with our Spiced Yogurt Sauce (page 231).

Meal: Main

Main Ingredients: Quinoa, Peppers

Prep Time: 30 minutes

Cook Time: 20 minutes

SERVES 4

4 poblano peppers

2 teaspoons extra-virgin olive oil for drizzling, divided

1½ cups panko or fine bread crumbs

1 teaspoon ground cumin

¾ cup grated Cotija or Parmesan cheese, divided

1½ cups cooked quinoa (see Basic Quinoa, page 33)

1½ cups grated cheddar

2 teaspoons crumbled dried oregano

Flour for dusting (see Ann's Tips, next page)

1 egg, beaten

1. Preheat the oven to broil.
2. Cover a broiling pan with aluminum foil. Place the peppers on the pan and place on the lowest rack of the broiler. Broil, turning occasionally, until the peppers' skin is blistered and charred all over. Place them in a brown paper bag (a supermarket bag is perfect), and loosely seal the top. Let steam in the bag for at least 10 minutes to loosen the skins.
3. Preheat the oven to 400°F. Line a baking sheet with parchment paper, drizzle with 1 teaspoon of the oil, and set aside.

4. Make the topping: In a medium bowl, mix the panko with the cumin and ¼ cup of the Cotija cheese. Sprinkle half the mixture on the prepared baking sheet and spread it out just long and wide enough to lay the peppers side by side with a half inch in between. Set the baking sheet aside. Reserve the remaining topping.

5. Make the filling: In a bowl, mix the cooked quinoa, the remaining ½ cup Cotija cheese, the cheddar cheese, and oregano. Stir until well blended. Set aside.

6. Rub or scrape the charred skins off the peppers—they should come off easily. Prepare them for stuffing. Keeping the top of the pepper intact, cut around the stalk end of the pepper until you have cut about halfway around the top. From the center of this cut, make a T shape by cutting down the length of the pepper. Gently open the pepper, and with a small, sharp knife, cut away the seeds and any white pith. Repeat with the remaining peppers. Divide the filling among the peppers. Close up the peppers so they look whole, and dust with flour.

7. Brush the cut side of each floured pepper with egg. Transfer the peppers seam-side down to the prepared baking sheet and lay atop the layer of seasoned panko. Leave a half inch between each. Brush more egg over the tops of the peppers. Without lifting them, gently rock each pepper from side to side to coat their bottom with panko. Sprinkle the tops and sides of the peppers with the remaining panko mixture a little at a time, pressing it in with your fingers as you go, until the peppers are well covered. Drizzle with the remaining 1 teaspoon oil. Bake on a rack set in the upper third of the oven for 15 to 20 minutes, or until the panko is lightly colored and the filling is hot and sticky. Serve immediately.

Ann's Tips

· ✳ ·

To make this dish gluten-free, use gluten-free bread crumbs and gluten-free garbanzo flour.

If you can't find poblanos, try either cubanelle or Italian frying peppers, and add ½ teaspoon of chili powder to the stuffing.

Brown rice or barley would be good substitutes here but quinoa is my favorite because of its short cooking time and complete protein content.

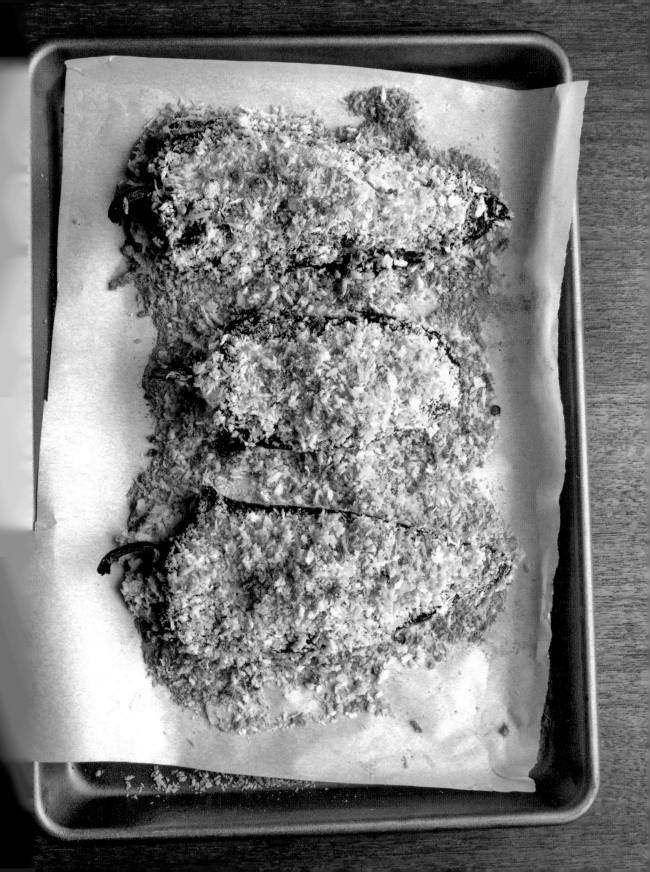

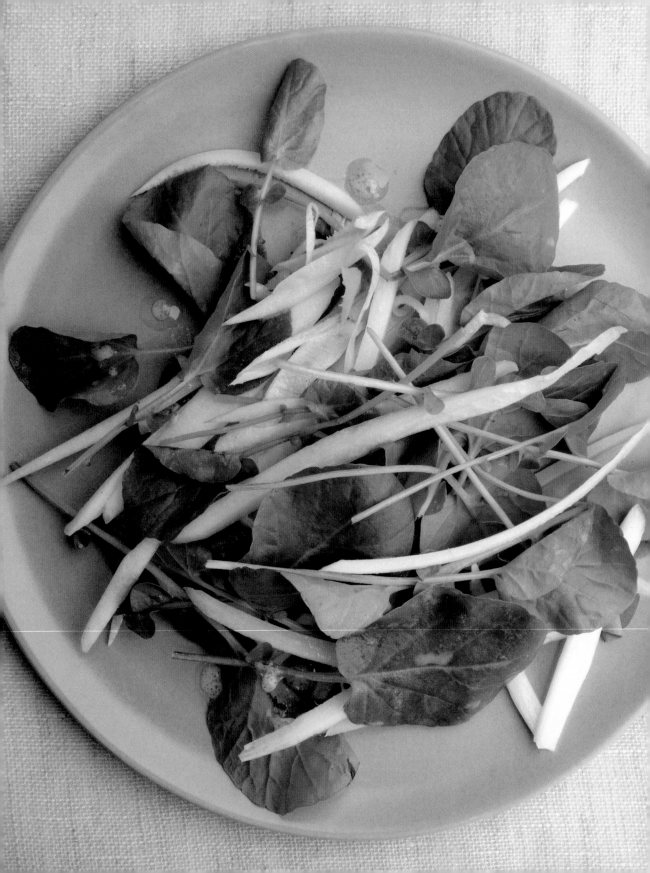

Belgian Endive and Watercress Salad

Meal: Salad

Main Ingredient: Endive, Watercress

Prep Time: 20 minutes

SERVES 4 TO 6

HEALTH CONSIDERATIONS: IN TREATMENT; FATIGUE; HIGH FIBER; GLUTEN-FREE; HEALTHY SURVIVORSHIP

FOOD PREFERENCE: DAIRY-FREE; VEGAN; VEGETARIAN

This winter favorite was a real treat to get back to after my doctors gave me the all-clear to eat raw foods again. I had missed this crunchy, mustardy salad more than I knew. Belgian endive is a vegetable worth getting to know. It is grown in the dark during the winter months, which keeps it white. What it may be lacking in color it makes up for in nutrition. It provides a treasure trove of different phytonutrients: vitamins A,C, K, and B complex, along with a good selection of minerals such as calcium, iron, zinc, copper, and more. What I love about this salad is the contrast in flavor between the juicy-sweet endive and the dark, almost bitter leaves of watercress, another super green from the A-list of healthy choices. And another excuse to enjoy this tangy, refreshing salad—not that I've ever needed one.

3 plump white Belgian endives

1 to 2 bunches watercress

Mustard Vinaigrette

1 tablespoon Dijon mustard

Sea salt and freshly ground black pepper, to taste

1½ tablespoons white wine vinegar

3 tablespoons extra-virgin olive oil

1 tablespoon cold water, or to taste

1. Quarter the endives and cut out the solid core. Slice them thinly lengthwise, transfer to a large colander, and rinse. Set aside.

2. Wash and dry the watercress in a salad spinner, or dry using a paper towel. Discard the thick, tough stems, putting only the slender branches of dark green leaves together with the shredded endive in the colander. Toss together to mix and set aside.
3. Make the vinaigrette: Spoon the mustard into a large salad bowl. Add a pinch of salt and a grind or two of black pepper. Using a small whisk, beat the vinegar into the mustard until it is completely blended and smooth.
4. Beating all the time, slowly add the oil into the mustard mixture until thoroughly combined and the mixture is smooth and creamy. Add ½ tablespoon of the water and beat to blend. Check for taste. If it is too strong, add the remaining ½ tablespoon water, or a little more oil, depending on how light you like your dressing.
5. Pile the endive and watercress on top of the dressing. Quickly toss together with the dressing when you are ready to eat.

Ann's Tips

Besides being great in salads, Belgian endive is also delicious braised, and the Italian red varieties are great browned on a hot grill, too.

Chicken Roasted in Cider

HEALTH CONSIDERATIONS: IN TREATMENT; FATIGUE; LOW FIBER; GLUTEN-FREE; NEUTROPENIC DIET; HEALTHY SURVIVORSHIP

FOOD PREFERENCE: DAIRY-FREE

Meal: Main

Main Ingredient: Chicken

Prep Time: 20 minutes

Cook Time: 90 minutes

SERVES 6

When I was a kid, my mom always used to serve applesauce with chicken. This is a more sophisticated-tasting way of combining apples and chicken, and is basically a cross between roasting and braising. The result is a moist chicken with tasty au jus gravy. The tart sweetness of the cider and the apples will also help counteract any taste changes treatment may have brought about, while simply tasting great to everyone else.

1 (3½- to 4-pound) organic free-range chicken

1 tablespoon extra-virgin olive oil, plus 2 teaspoons for drizzling

1½ cups hard dry cider, divided (see Ann's Tips, next page)

Sea salt, to taste

3 tart apples, halved and cores scooped out

1. Preheat the oven to 500°F with a heavy roasting pan placed on a center rack.
2. Remove the packet of giblets from the chicken and tie the legs together with twine (optional). Rub the chicken all over with 1 tablespoon of the oil. Remove the hot roasting pan from the oven and drizzle with the remaining oil. Transfer the chicken to the pan and roast for 20 minutes.
3. Lower the heat to 350°F. Remove the pan from the oven. Add ¾ cup of cider to the hot pan, sprinkle the chicken with salt, and return to the oven. Roast for 35 minutes, basting from time to time, adding cider by the quarter cup if the pan looks dry.
4. Add the apples to the pan, cut-sides down, plus another ¼ cup of cider. Roast another 25 minutes, basting the bird from time to time. Turn the apples over

and roast 20 minutes more, or until the chicken is cooked or a meat thermometer stuck between the breast and the drumstick reads 160°F.

5. Let the bird sit for 10 minutes before carving. Deglaze the pan with the remaining cider and let it bubble. Transfer the pan juices into a fat-separating jug, if you have one. If you don't have one, tilt the pan and spoon off as much of the golden fat from the top of the gravy juices as you can. Pour the remaining pan juices into a gravy boat to serve with the carved chicken.

Ann's Tips

· ✳ ·

If you can't find hard dry cider, use a nonalcoholic clear sparkling cider such as Martinelli's.

This dish is very simple, so buy the best-quality chicken you can afford. When roasting, chicken usually needs 15 minutes per pound, with an additional 15 minutes cooking time tacked on at the end to get the right doneness. With this recipe, since most of the time the oven is a little cooler than usual, for a 4-pound bird I've added an extra 5 minutes per pound.

Adding the chicken's giblets sprinkled with salt to the body cavity adds a lot of flavor, with the exception of the liver. The liver can get bitter if overcooked, so reserve it for another use.

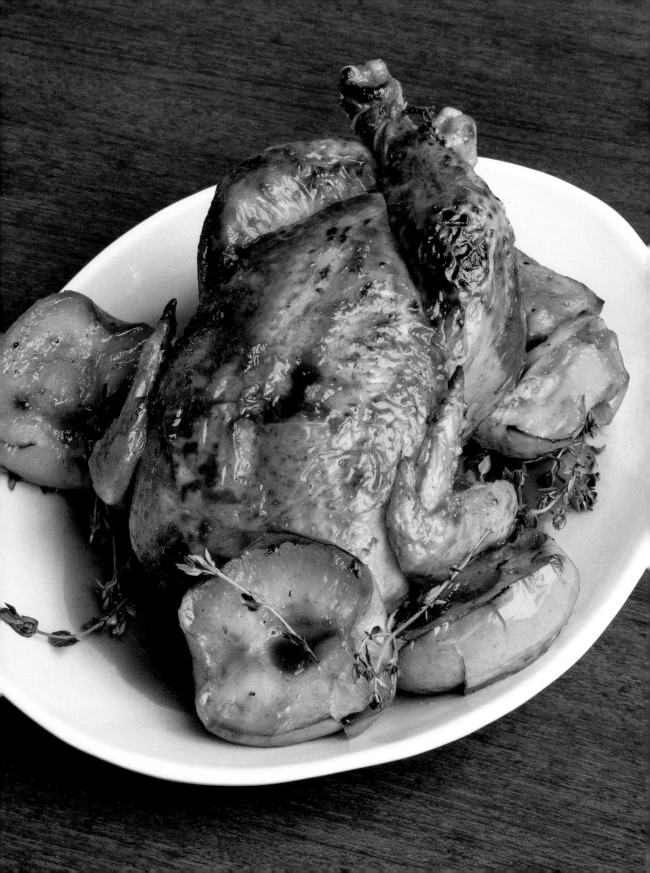

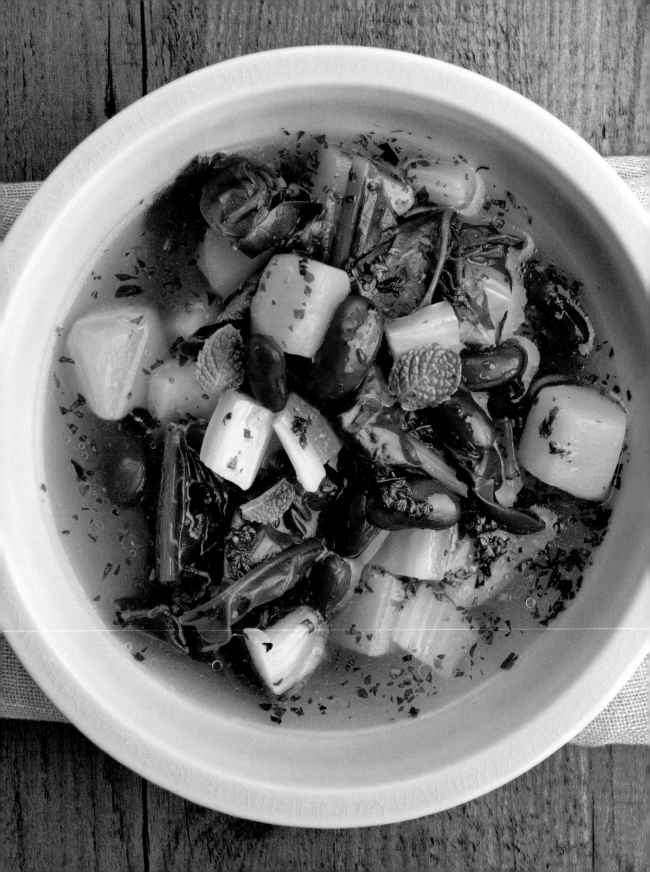

Fall Market Soup with Dukkah

HEALTH CONSIDERATIONS: IN TREATMENT; HIGH FIBER; GLUTEN-FREE; NEUTROPENIC DIET; HEALTHY SURVIVORSHIP

FOOD PREFERENCE: DAIRY-FREE; VEGAN; VEGETARIAN

This delicious winter soup is a nutritious temptation for a cold winter's day. Two of my favorite winter market vegetables are there: orange butternut squash, and pale fennel. The soup's rich earthiness comes from dark green chard leaves, brightened by the sharpness of lemon, and aromatic dukkah paste. This combo is the perfect antidote to a jaded chemo palate. It's also easy to make. If your energy is low, use all the conveniences that supermarket produce sections offer to save on prep time: peeled garlic, peeled and precut squash, and canned beans. And it's a big soup, so you'll have plenty for the freezer to whip up a tasty quick supper when you don't feel like cooking.

> **Meal:** Soup
>
> **Main Ingredients:** Butternut squash, Chard, Kidney beans
>
> **Prep Time:** 30 minutes
>
> **Cook Time:** 35 minutes
>
> **SERVES 8 TO 10**

2 tablespoons extra-virgin olive oil

1 medium yellow onion, diced

1 small fennel bulb, diced

6 cups butternut squash, cut into 1-inch dice

1 bay leaf

Zest and juice of 1 medium lemon

2 cloves garlic, peeled and smashed

Sea salt and freshly ground black pepper, to taste

6 cups water (see Ann's Tips, next page)

2 cans dark red kidney beans, rinsed and drained, or 1 recipe Basic Beans #1 (page 38) (see Ann's Tips, next page)

3 cups Swiss chard leaves, torn into bite-size pieces (see Ann's Tips, next page)

Lemon wedges, for garnish

Dukkah Paste

3 sprigs mint, leaves stripped

1 sprig tarragon, leaves stripped (optional)

½ teaspoon cumin seeds

½ teaspoon sea salt

2 teaspoons extra-virgin olive oil

1. Heat the oil over medium-high heat in a large Dutch oven. When hot, add the onion, fennel, squash, and bay leaf. Cook, stirring occasionally, 5 to 8 minutes, or until the onion becomes translucent. Add the lemon zest and garlic. Sprinkle with salt and stir to mix. Lower the heat to medium-low, cover, and gently cook the vegetables for 8 to 10 minutes, stirring from time to time, or until the onion and fennel are soft and the squash is beginning to soften.

2. Add the water and bring the soup to a low boil. Cover, lower the heat, and simmer for 20 minutes, or until the squash is just tender but not falling apart.

3. While the soup is cooking, make the dukkah paste: Roughly chop the mint and tarragon, if using, then add the cumin and salt. Chop everything together. When roughly blended, very gradually add the oil and chop into a paste on the cutting board. Set aside in a small bowl.

4. Add the red beans to the soup. If they are homemade, add the cooking broth, too. Bring to a simmer and cook for 15 minutes. Add the chard leaves in two to three batches, adding another as each batch wilts into the soup. When all the chard has been added, cook for 5 minutes, or until completely soft. Stir in the lemon juice and the dukkah paste. Cook for 2 minutes more. Serve hot with lemon wedges.

Ann's Tips

· ✶ ·

The red kidney beans in this soup are the deep dark red variety used in Italian cooking and not Spanish red kidney beans, also called coloradas, that are, in fact, pink.

When freezing, add the lemon juice and dukkah to the soup once it's thawed. If that's a hassle, freeze the soup with everything added, and cut a little wedge of lemon to squeeze over your bowl just before eating.

Beet Risotto

HEALTH CONSIDERATIONS: IN TREATMENT; EASY TO SWALLOW; BLAND DIET; HIGH FIBER; GLUTEN-FREE; NEUTROPENIC DIET; HEALTHY SURVIVORSHIP

FOOD PREFERENCE: VEGETARIAN

Meal: Main

Main Ingredients: Beets, Arborio rice

Prep Time: 20 minutes

Cook Time: 30 minutes

SERVES 4

This gorgeously rich, deep-crimson risotto moves beets from the ordinary to the sublime. Most of this nutritious vegetable, from its sweet earthy roots to the tips of its deep green leaves, goes into this satisfying dish. And although the recipe calls for just 2 beets, you can use all the greens from the bunch. I won't deny that hand grating beets is a messy job. I always feel like Lady Macbeth when I've finished, with more than a few damn spots to get out. However, if you have a food processor, the grating tool provides a speedier, less messy solution. And there's always gloves. Whichever way you choose to attack the beets, you'll find the final results well worth the effort.

2 large beets with their greens (about ½ bunch) (see Ann's Tips, next page)

1 tablespoon extra-virgin olive oil

1 medium onion, diced

½ teaspoon dried thyme or 1½ teaspoons fresh thyme

½ teaspoon grated lemon zest

Sea salt, to taste

1 cup arborio rice

¼ cup dry white wine

4 cups Basic Vegetable Broth (page 21) or Quick, Rich Chicken Broth (page 24), kept warm on the stove

3 tablespoons grated Parmesan cheese, plus extra for serving

1 tablespoon unsalted butter

1. Cut the leaves off the beets. If they are fresh and in good condition, wash, destem, and shred the leaves. Set aside. Discard the stems.
2. Trim and scrub the beets—you don't need to peel them. Grate coarsely, using a box grater or food processor. Set aside.

3. In a large Dutch oven, heat the oil over medium-high heat. Add the onion, thyme, and lemon zest. Cook until the onion becomes translucent, about 3 minutes. Add beets, sprinkle with salt, and cook, stirring, for 5 minutes.

4. Add the rice and cook, stirring, for 5 minutes, or until the rice starts to absorb the oil and beet juices. Add the white wine. Cook until completely absorbed by the rice. Add the broth, ½ cup at a time, and cook, stirring, until each addition is absorbed. Repeat with all but 1 cup of the stock.

5. Add the cheese, butter, shredded greens, and ½ cup of the remaining broth. Stir until the liquid looks creamy. Cover. Turn off the heat and leave to sit for 5 minutes. Taste for salt. The dish should have a creamy consistency, so if the rice looks thick and sticky, stir in the remaining stock to reach the desired consistency. Serve immediately.

Ann's Tips

· ⚶ ·

The sizes of bunches of beets found at the supermarket can vary wildly, but average 4 beets plus their greens. As noted in the introduction, you can use all the greens from the bunch.

Creamy goat cheese and beets are a marriage made in heaven. In step 5, instead of the Parmesan, stir in 1 tablespoon of soft goat cheese.

If you aren't strictly vegetarian, use chicken broth for this.

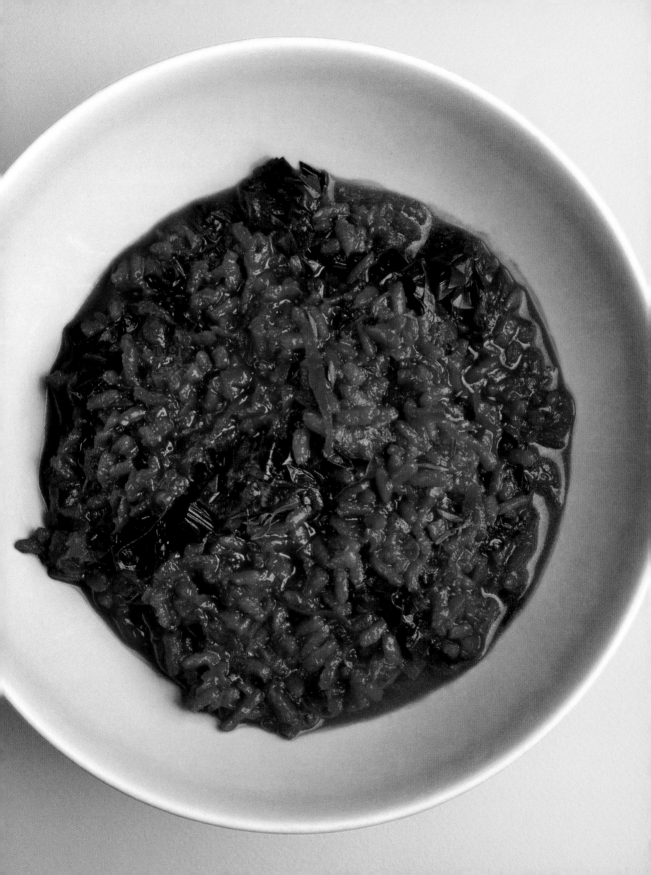

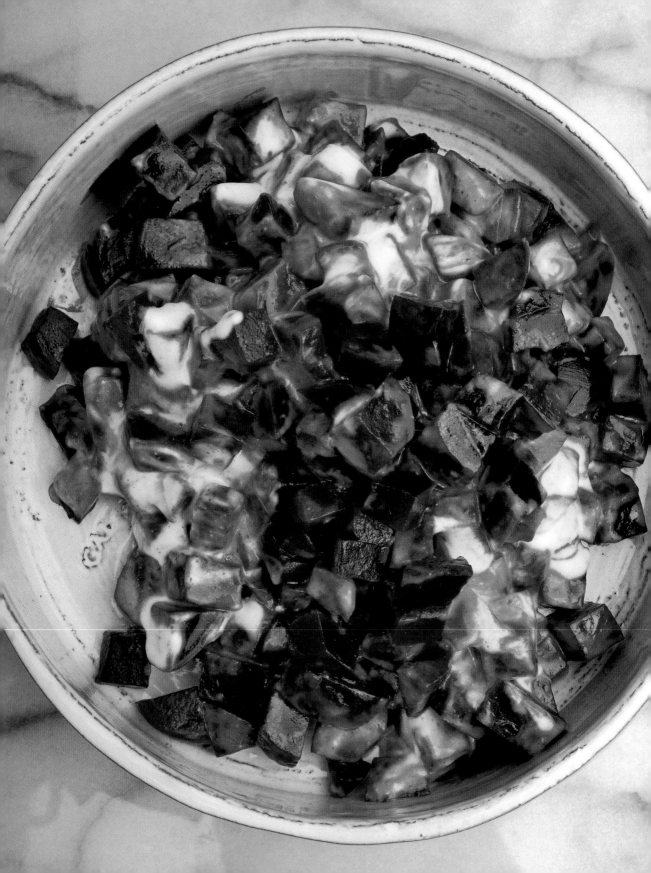

Baltic Beet Salad

HEALTH CONSIDERATIONS: GLUTEN-FREE; IN TREATMENT; HEALTHY SURVIVORSHIP; NEUTROPENIC DIET

FOOD PREFERENCE: VEGETARIAN

Meal: Side

Main Ingredient: Beets

Prep Time: 15 minutes

Cook Time: 40 minutes

SERVES 4

Roasted beets are candy-sweet. This Baltic-inspired dish is a wonderfully simple way to use them to make a really excellent salad either as a starter or a side dish, and I love it as a condiment in sandwiches. Roasting beets doesn't demand a lot of energy, but you do need time, so if that's something you don't have, use vacuum-packed beets. They are simply steamed without vinegar, and just need to be drained before use. Although not as sweet as roasted beets, vacuum-packed beets are good, extremely convenient, and—since they don't need refrigeration until they are opened—a great pantry item.

Health Tip

If you are following a neutropenic diet, check with your doctor or registered dietitian to determine if yogurt is within your dietary guidelines.

---

1 bunch red beets (about 4 beets), washed and trimmed (greens reserved for another use) (see Ann's Tips, next page)

¼ cup extra-virgin olive oil, plus extra for brushing

1 clove garlic, smashed (optional)

1 tablespoon cider vinegar

1 tablespoon Dijon mustard

Sea salt and freshly ground black pepper, to taste

2 tablespoons whole-milk or 2% plain Greek yogurt

1 tablespoon water, as needed

1. Preheat the oven to 375°F.
2. Halve the beets and brush with a little oil, then wrap each half in foil. Put on a

baking sheet and bake for 35 to 40 minutes, or until the beets are soft. The length of time they take will depend on their size.

3. While the beets are baking, rub the bottom and sides of a medium ceramic serving bowl with the smashed garlic, if using. (This will add a hint of garlic to the salad.) In a separate bowl, whisk together the vinegar, mustard, and salt and pepper. Gradually whisk in the ¼ cup of oil, then the yogurt until smooth. Taste for sharpness and seasoning. Add water, 1 teaspoon at a time, if the dressing tastes too sharp.

4. When the beets are cooked and cool enough to handle but still warm, rub the skins off and cut them into small dice. Throw them into the prepared salad bowl and stir. Spoon the dressing over the beets 1 tablespoon at a time, tossing the beets as you go, until the beets are just covered with dressing but not swimming in it. Save any extra dressing for another salad. Serve as a side or starter.

Ann's Tips
· ✳ ·

All parts of raw red beets will stain your hands once you've cut them, leaves included. When handling beets, either use gloves or wash your hands with soap directly after coming into contact with their juices. That said, beets are nutrient packed, delicious, and totally worth the trouble.

Vacuum-packed beets are becoming easier to find. Look locally for Melissa's, Rocal, Whole Foods 365 brand beets, or Trader Joe's steamed and peeled baby beets.

Autumnal Roasted Vegetable Salad

Meal: Side, Salad

Main Ingredients: Beets, Winter squash, Sweet potatoes, Rutabaga

Prep Time: 40 minutes

Cook Time: 45 minutes

SERVES 4 TO 6

HEALTH CONSIDERATIONS: IN TREATMENT; BLAND DIET; GLUTEN-FREE; HEALTHY SURVIVORSHIP; NEUTROPENIC DIET

FOOD PREFERENCE: DAIRY-FREE; VEGETARIAN

This great salad can use any fall veggies. Here we've taken golden beets, squash, sweet potatoes, and even rutabaga, roasted them and tossed them in a pomegranate vinaigrette. Roasting transforms vegetables. Although gnarly but nutritious, rutabaga requires a little parboiling to soften it up, but once in the roasting pan, it finds its inner sweetness. The sharp taste of the pomegranate dressing offsets the rich taste of these roasted vegetables to perfection. This salad is gorgeous to look at, delicious to eat, and good for you.

1 medium rutabaga, cut into 1-inch dice

2 medium (or 1 large) golden beets, cut into 1-inch wedges

1 small butternut or acorn squash, peeled and cut into 1-inch dice

2 medium red sweet potatoes, peeled and cut into 1-inch dice

1 tablespoon extra-virgin olive oil

2 shallots, peeled and thinly sliced

2 tablespoons pomegranate seeds (optional)

2 tablespoons sliced almonds, toasted (page 48)

Pomegranate Vinaigrette

1 tablespoon apple cider vinegar or water

1 teaspoon honey

Sea salt and freshly ground black pepper, to taste

2 tablespoons pomegranate molasses (see Ann's Tips, page 307)

¼ cup plus 1 tablespoon extra-virgin olive oil

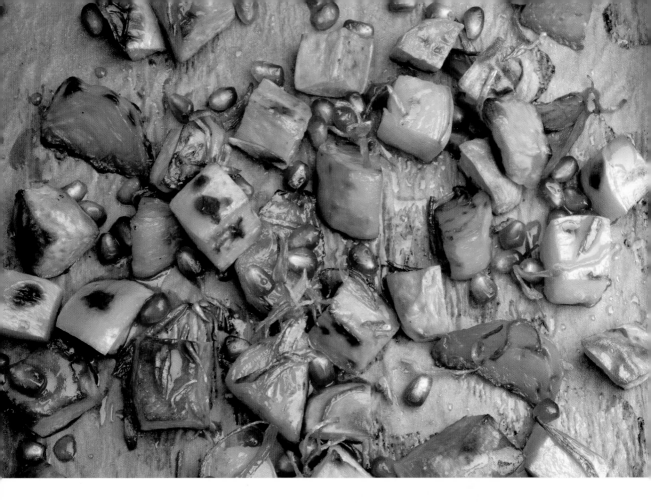

1. Preheat the oven to 400°F. Line a baking sheet with parchment paper and set aside.

2. Bring a large pan of water to a boil. Add the rutabaga to the pan and cook for 10 minutes. Drain and pat dry.

3. In a large bowl, toss the beets, squash, sweet potatoes, and rutabaga with the oil and spread the vegetables in a single layer on the prepared baking sheet. Toss the shallots in the oil remaining in the bowl and set aside.

4. Roast the vegetables on a rack in the upper third of the oven for 15 minutes. Remove the vegetables from the oven and turn them. Add the shallots to the baking sheet and roast for 30 to 35 minutes longer, or until vegetables are tender and slightly caramelized.

5. Make the vinaigrette: In a large salad bowl, whisk the vinegar, honey, salt and pepper, and pomegranate molasses until completely smooth. Whisking continuously, slowly add the oil until you have an even, thick dressing. Taste for sharpness; if it is too sharp, add a little cold water or oil depending on how heavy you like your dressing. Set aside.

6. When the vegetables are cooked, transfer them to the bowl with the dressing and toss to mix. Allow to rest for at least 30 minutes, or until ready to serve. The longer the vegetables marinate in the dressing, the better they will taste. Do not refrigerate.

7. Before serving, toss in the pomegranate seeds, if using, and pile the vegetables onto a large serving plate. Sprinkle with the almonds. Serve warm or at room temperature.

Ann's Tips

Because vegetables aren't uniform in shape and size, it's difficult to make them exactly the same size for even cooking, so cooking times are approximate. Some are tender, like winter squash, and may need less cooking, while others, like rutabaga, are a little harder and need parboiling to soften so the rest of the vegetables don't overcook.

You can find pomegranate molasses in Middle Eastern groceries or the international section of many supermarkets, and, failing that, Amazon. Use Saba balsamic syrup as a substitute.

This dish stores and travels well and can therefore be a delicious way to keep vegetables on hand. Other vegetables can be roasted with this method. I like to make a batch and incorporate the veggies in multiple meals throughout the week.

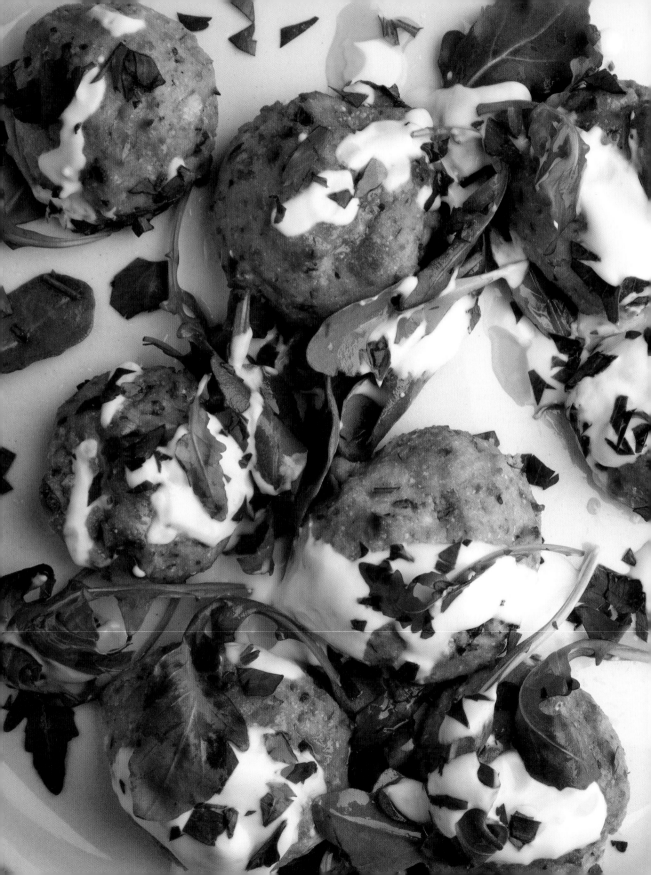

Eggplant Polpettone

HEALTH CONSIDERATIONS: IN TREATMENT; HIGH FIBER; GLUTEN-FREE
(SEE ANN'S TIPS NEXT PAGE); NEUTROPENIC DIET; HEALTHY SURVIVORSHIP

FOOD PREFERENCE: VEGETARIAN

Meal: Main

Main Ingredients: Eggplant, Ricotta

Prep Time: 30 minutes

Cook Time: 45 minutes

MAKES ABOUT 20 TO 24 "MEATBALLS" (SERVES 3 TO 4)

These vegetarian eggplant "meatballs" are absolutely delicious, and versatile, too. Baked instead of fried, they can be used as a super-light substitute in almost any dish that calls for meat. The mix can even be baked like a meat loaf. Try them as an appetizer dipped in Greek yogurt drizzled with good olive oil, or on a salad of dark greens, or as a crowd-pleaser over pasta, tossed with Quick Tomato Sauce (page 27). They're good every which way.

2 medium Italian eggplants

½ cup ricotta cheese

1 egg, lightly beaten

1 tablespoon extra-virgin olive oil, plus more for drizzling

¾ teaspoon sea salt

1 tablespoon chopped fresh rosemary, stems removed

2 large cloves garlic, minced

Freshly ground black pepper, to taste (optional)

½ cup almond flour

1 cup whole-wheat bread crumbs, or gluten-free bread crumbs (see Ann's Tips, next page)

6 tablespoons grated Pecorino cheese, or to taste

1. Preheat the oven to broil. Cover a broiling pan with aluminum foil and set aside.
2. Cut the stalk end off the eggplants and score them a couple of times down each side. Transfer to the prepared broiling pan on a low shelf under the broiler and broil, turning from time to time, about 30 minutes or until they are soft and the skin is charred all over. Set aside to cool. Lower the oven temperature to 400°F.
3. Once the eggplants are cool enough to handle, scrape the flesh out onto a cutting board and finely chop, making sure not to get any charred skin in the flesh.
4. Line a baking sheet with parchment paper and drizzle with oil. Set aside.

5. In a large bowl, using a whisk, mix the eggplant, ricotta, egg, oil, salt, rosemary, garlic, and a grind or two of black pepper, if using, until well combined and smooth.

6. With a spatula or a wooden spoon, fold in the almond flour, bread crumbs, and Pecorino until you have a stiff yet soft and sticky paste. Using your hands, roll the mixture into 1-inch balls and arrange them in a single layer on the prepared baking sheet.

7. Bake for 15 minutes on the center rack of the oven. Turn the balls over and bake for 10 minutes more, or until they are completely golden. Serve as desired.

Ann's Tips

· ✻ ·

Instead of broiling the eggplant, you can either cook it on the grill or place it on a hot baking sheet and bake at 450°F in the upper third of the oven.

For gluten-free, use your favorite gluten-free bread or bread crumbs. To make your own bread crumbs, cube stale whole-grain bread (I use the leftover heels), and pulse in the food processor until fine crumbs form. Store leftovers in the freezer, where they will keep indefinitely.

Buckwheat Noodle Casserole with Ricotta and Sage Butter

Meal: Main

Main Ingredients: Soba noodles, Cabbage

Prep Time: 20 minutes

Cook Time: 30 minutes

SERVES 6 TO 8

HEALTH CONSIDERATIONS: IN TREATMENT; EASY TO SWALLOW; FATIGUE; HIGH FIBER; NEUTROPENIC DIET

FOOD PREFERENCE: VEGETARIAN

This is a version of a Northern Italian cold-weather dish that is one of the tastiest cabbage dishes I know of. It's traditionally made with savoy cabbage cooked in brown butter, cheese, and a regional buckwheat pasta called *pizzoccheri*. Our version still makes the "naughty but nice" cut because it is high in saturated fat thanks to that brown butter. But there's enough good here, thanks to the sweet savoy cabbage and light ricotta cheese, to make this a great replacement for the occasional mac 'n' cheese. *Pizzoccheri* are not easy to come by, but soba noodles are. Although not as chunky as the original, their flavor is right and they make an excellent substitute in this delicious, comforting, stick-to-your-ribs meal.

5 tablespoons unsalted butter, divided

2 cloves garlic, divided; 1 peeled and smashed, 1 minced

8 leaves fresh sage, divided; 4 whole and 4 minced

8 ounces soba or buckwheat noodles

2 leeks, whites only, julienned (see Ann's Tips, page 313)

Sea salt, to taste

10 cups savoy cabbage, quartered, cored, and thinly sliced into ¼-inch strips

½ cup freshly grated Parmesan cheese

1 cup whole-wheat bread crumbs

½ cup grated Gruyère

1½ cups ricotta cheese

1. Make the brown butter: Melt 4 tablespoons of the butter in a small saucepan over medium-low heat (see Ann's Tips, page 313). Add the smashed garlic clove

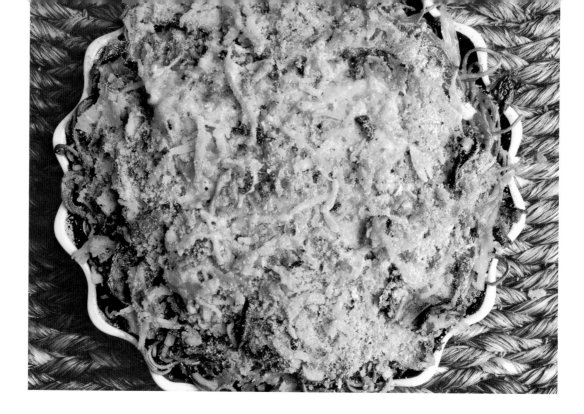

and 4 whole sage leaves. The butter will foam and turn a lemony yellow. Continue to cook slowly until the garlic is golden, the sage leaves are crisp, and the butter is a toasty brown, about 15 minutes. Discard the garlic if it gets too dark. Strain through a fine sieve or cheesecloth into a bowl and set aside, reserving the sage leaves.

2. Set a large pan of salted water to boil. Cook the soba noodles 2 minutes short of the recommended package cooking time. Drain noodles, reserving 1 cup of the cooking water, and rinse. Toss the noodles in half the brown butter. Set aside.

3. Preheat the oven to 425°F. Grease a 2-quart ceramic baking dish and set aside.

4. Heat the remaining brown butter in a sauté pan over medium-high heat. Add the minced garlic and minced sage leaves and cook until the garlic begins to color, about 1 minute. Add the leeks, sprinkle with salt, and cook, stirring until they start to soften, about 3 minutes. Add 5 cups of the cabbage, sprinkle with salt, and cook, stirring, until it starts to wilt, then add the rest, stirring to mix,

about 10 minutes. As soon as that wilts, too, add 2 tablespoons of the pasta cooking water, cover the pan, and reduce the heat to low. Cook until the cabbage is soft, about 10 minutes. Add another 2 tablespoons of the pasta cooking water if the cabbage looks dry. Stir in the Parmesan cheese and cook until it melts into the cabbage.

5. To assemble the dish: Mix the bread crumbs and the Gruyère together and crumble in the butter-cooked sage leaves. Set aside. Put half the soba noodles in the prepared baking dish. Cover with about two-thirds of the vegetables, then spread the ricotta over the vegetables. Add the rest of the soba and finish with the remaining vegetables. Cover the top with the bread crumb mixture. Dot with the remaining 1 tablespoon butter. Bake for 15 to 20 minutes, or until the top is crisp and golden. Serve piping-hot.

Ann's Tips

· ✈ ·

The flavor of the brown butter is an integral part of this dish. Brown butter is delicious and has so many uses in the kitchen. It is great with simply cooked fish or to add flavor to sautés, but I am particularly fond of it cooked with sage leaves as a sauce for pumpkin ravioli or to drizzle over pumpkin soup. Brown butter is basically ghee. It has a high smoke point and will keep indefinitely in the fridge once you've made it. The trick is to cook it very slowly so you don't burn it. I don't recommend using a skillet, even a small one, as the butter will cook too fast and burn. Use a small saucepan, light-colored if you have one, so you can see the color change. As you cook it, once the butter has stopped foaming, you will notice some sediment has formed in the pan that gets darker as the butter cooks. This is normal. Butter has a lot of moisture that gets cooked out of it, leaving the milk solids as sediment. This is what burns if the butter cooks too fast. The brown butter is ready when it's a rich golden-brown color, you can smell its nuttiness, and the sediment is a deep red-brown. Strain the butter through a fine-mesh strainer or cheesecloth before either storing or using.

Although this dish tastes plenty cheesy, if you prefer a more melted cheese experience than ricotta on its own will give, mix ½ cup of grated mozzarella cheese in with 1 cup of ricotta.

Salt-Grilled Tofu with Citrus Remoulade Sauce

Meal: Main

Main Ingredient: Tofu

Prep Time: 10 minutes, plus 30 minutes resting time

Cook Time: 10 minutes

SERVES 4

HEALTH CONSIDERATIONS: IN TREATMENT; EASY TO SWALLOW; LOW FIBER; GLUTEN-FREE; NEUTROPENIC DIET; HEALTHY SURVIVORSHIP

FOOD PREFERENCE: DAIRY-FREE; VEGAN; VEGETARIAN; NUTS

A lot of people say they don't like tofu because it has no taste. Not so with this dish. Salting makes tofu really delicious when grilled, and the smooth sauce with its citrusy tang is a terrific foil to its natural mildness. Served with some steamed greens and rice, this recipe is a lovely way to turn tofu into a tasty treat for a perfect light lunch or dinner. It is important to get as much water out of the tofu as possible, so don't skip the draining step (see Ann's Tips, next page). Wet tofu tends to stick to the grill. The sauce is a keeper, too, a delicious condiment that will liven up any simply cooked vegetables, fish, or chicken.

1 (16-ounce) block of firm or extra-firm tofu, cut into 1-inch-thick slices

1 to 2 teaspoons sea salt

1 teaspoon peanut oil

Citrus Remoulade Sauce

1 tablespoon tahini

1 tablespoon Dijon mustard

1 tablespoon apple cider vinegar

1 tablespoon lemon juice

3 tablespoons extra-virgin olive oil

2 tablespoons water

Sea salt and freshly ground black pepper, to taste

1. Drain the tofu: Line a tray with paper towels and place the tofu slices on top in a single layer. Cover with more paper towels and top with a heavy cutting board to act as a weight. Place one end of the tray close to the edge of the sink and

raise the back end slightly with a spoon or a book. Let drain for 30 to 40 minutes. You will be amazed at how much water comes out.

2. While the tofu is draining, make the sauce: Whisk the tahini and the mustard together until well blended. Whisk in the vinegar, lemon juice, then the oil, a little at a time. Whisk in the water as needed until you have a thick sauce. Taste for salt and pepper. Set aside.

3. Preheat a grill pan over medium-high heat.

4. Pat the drained tofu slices dry. Dampen your index and middle fingers and dip into the salt. Take a tofu slice and rub all sides with the salt. Set aside. Repeat until all the slices have been salted.

5. Brush the hot grill with the oil and grill the tofu slices without crowding, in batches if necessary. Cook the slices for 4 to 5 minutes, then, using a spatula, flip them over. They will be covered with brown grill marks. Grill the other side for 4 minutes more, or until browned. Keep them warm while you grill the remaining slices. Eat hot, drizzled with the remoulade sauce.

Ann's Tips

Draining tofu is a good trick to know. It helps marinated or stir-fried tofu absorb more flavor. For marinades, slice and drain as directed, and for stir-fries, slice the block of tofu in half horizontally to form 2 thinner slices the same length and width as the original block and drain as directed before using.

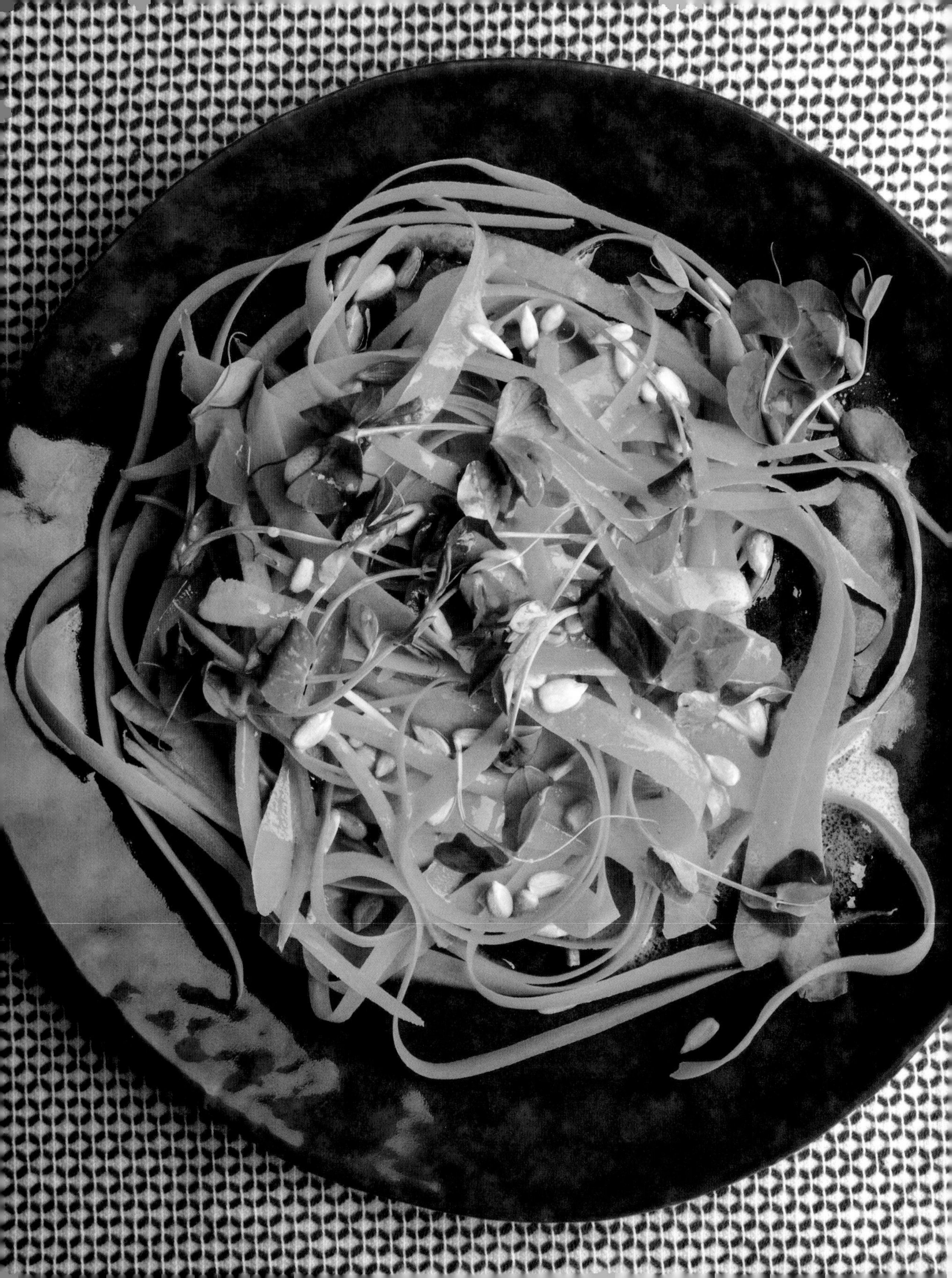

Carrot Ribbon Salad

HEALTH CONSIDERATIONS: FATIGUE; NAUSEA; HIGH FIBER; GLUTEN-FREE; HEALTHY SURVIVORSHIP

FOOD PREFERENCE: DAIRY-FREE; VEGAN; VEGETARIAN

Meal: Salad

Main Ingredient: Carrots

Prep Time: 15 minutes

SERVES 4

This is a great way to use large carrots with woody cores. Their sweetness is wonderful with toasty sunflower seeds and salty-sweet *shiro* (white) miso. *Shiro* miso is a great pantry item. You can use it in dressings, as in this recipe, or to flavor soups and stews. Kept in the fridge, it lasts indefinitely.

Sunflower sprouts are crunchy, delicious, and chock-full of phytonutrients. If you can't find them, pea shoots or arugula are a great substitute.

Health Tip

Miso is a fermented soy product and a probiotic, containing live microorganisms that can help keep your gut flora healthy. If you have had a stem cell transplant, however, your doctor may not allow you to eat any probiotics at all, including miso. Check with your health-care team before consuming miso.

2 large carrots, scrubbed well

1 tablespoon *shiro* (white) miso (see Ann's Tips, next page)

1 tablespoon lemon juice

1 tablespoon water

½ teaspoon agave syrup (optional)

1 tablespoon extra-virgin olive oil

2 tablespoons shelled raw sunflower seeds, dry-toasted (page 48)

1 cup sunflower sprouts or pea shoots, rinsed

1. Starting with one carrot, use a peeler to make a thin ribbon by shaving the carrot down its length, top to bottom. Keep cutting, turning the carrot after each

stroke, until you are left with the woody core and a pile of carrot ribbons. Discard the core and repeat with the other carrot. Set the ribbons aside.

2. In a large bowl, whisk together the *shiro* miso, lemon juice, water, and agave syrup, if using, until smooth. Whisk in the oil. Add more water, 1 teaspoon at a time, if the dressing is too thick. Pile the carrots and toasted sunflower seeds on top of the dressing and toss together. Just before you are ready to serve the salad, pile the sunflower sprouts on top and toss together with the carrots.

Ann's Tips

·✻·

White miso can usually be found at Asian markets, or in the supermarket with tofu and other soy products.

Roasted Green Beans with Chopping Board Pesto

Meal: Side

Main Ingredient: Green beans

Prep Time: 10 minutes

Cook Time: 10 minutes

SERVES 4

HEALTH CONSIDERATIONS: IN TREATMENT; FATIGUE; HIGH FIBER; GLUTEN-FREE; HEALTHY SURVIVORSHIP

FOOD PREFERENCE: DAIRY-FREE; VEGAN; VEGETARIAN

Green beans are wonderful roasted. Take care not to overcook them—you want them caramelized but not burned. Chopping board pesto is a quick and easy way to make small amounts of pesto to season soups and basic vegetables without using a food processor or mortar and pestle. All you need is a chef's knife to combine and chop the ingredients together. It's totally marvelous with these beans. Try it.

3 tablespoons extra-virgin olive oil, or as needed, divided

1 pound green beans, trimmed (see Ann's Tips, next page)

1 teaspoon sea salt, or to taste, divided

1 to 2 cloves garlic, or to taste, peeled

3 sprigs fresh basil, leaves stripped

1. Preheat the oven to 425°F and warm a large baking sheet in the top third of the oven while the oven is heating. Cut a piece of parchment paper to fit the baking sheet. Set aside.
2. Place 1 tablespoon of the oil in a large bowl. Add the green beans, sprinkle with a little salt, and toss until the beans are lightly coated. Set aside.
3. On a clean chopping board, slice the garlic, and chop it with a chef's knife. When it is roughly chopped, sprinkle with ½ teaspoon of the salt and chop it in. Add the basil leaves and chop them into the garlic and salt. When the basil is chopped quite fine, add a little more salt and drizzle in the oil, a little at a time,

until you have a soft, aromatic paste. Scrape it off the board and into a serving bowl. Taste for salt.

4. Pull the hot sheet from the oven and quickly cover with the reserved parchment paper. Transfer the green beans onto the hot sheet in one layer. Turn them when they have softened and have begun to caramelize on one side, 8 to 10 minutes. Roast another 5 to 8 minutes, or until the beans have softened and have caramelized patches all over.

5. Tip in the hot beans into the pesto and quickly toss to coat. Serve immediately.

Ann's Tips

· ✻ ·

To get the most benefits from garlic's cancer-fighting properties, once it's been cut or chopped, let it rest 5 to 10 minutes before using.

You can grill the beans, too. At home I cook them on a cast-iron grill pan, but if I'm outside, I put them on the barbecue, loosely wrapped in foil so that they don't fall onto the coals.

If you like cheese, stir 1 tablespoon of freshly grated Pecorino Romano cheese into the pesto just before you add the beans in step 4.

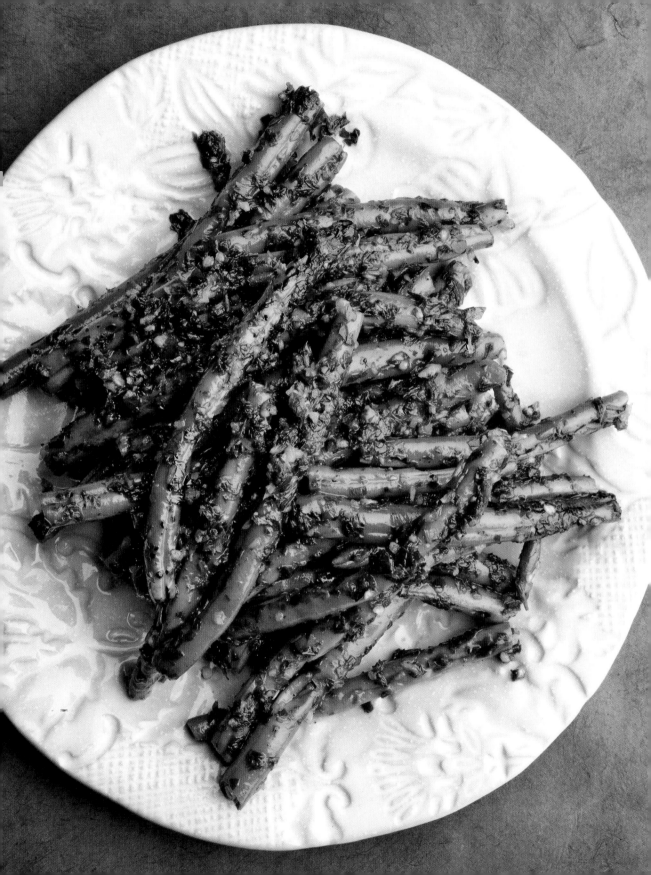

Buckwheat Pancakes with Peaches and Blueberries

Meal: Breakfast

Main Ingredients:
Buckwheat, Buttermilk

Prep Time: 15 minutes

Cook Time: 20 minutes

SERVES 3 TO 4

HEALTH CONSIDERATIONS: IN TREATMENT; EASY TO SWALLOW; NAUSEA; BLAND DIET; HIGH FIBER; HEALTHY SURVIVORSHIP

FOOD PREFERENCE: VEGETARIAN

Fresh summer fruit tossed with just a little maple syrup for flavor is a mouthwatering substitute for sloshing neat maple syrup over pancakes. Delicious as it is, maple syrup is pure sugar, but mixed with fruit, as it is here, it makes a healthier topping for these tasty, almost savory buckwheat pancakes.

1 large ripe peach, or 2 small peaches, washed, skinned, and diced (see Ann's Tips, next page)

1 cup fresh blueberries, washed

1 tablespoon maple syrup

1 teaspoon water

¼ cup unbleached all-purpose or whole-wheat pastry flour

¾ cup buckwheat flour

½ teaspoon baking powder

¼ teaspoon baking soda

1 tablespoon brown sugar

¼ teaspoon sea salt

1 cup plus 2 tablespoons buttermilk

1 large egg, lightly beaten

1 tablespoon butter, melted, plus 1 teaspoon for the skillet

1. Mix the peaches, blueberries, maple syrup, and water together and set aside in a cool place to macerate. If the mixture seems dry, add another teaspoon of water. The fruit will create juice as it sits, so don't add too much liquid.
2. In a medium bowl, whisk together the flours, baking powder, baking soda, sugar, and salt. Make a well in the center and stir in the buttermilk, egg, and 1 tablespoon of melted butter with a wooden spoon or a silicone spatula, just until combined. Allow the batter to rest for 5 minutes.

3. Heat a heavy skillet or nonstick pan over medium heat until hot. Brush with a little butter—you don't need too much. Wipe off any excess with a paper towel and reserve for your next batch.

4. Using a ¼-cup ladle, spoon the batter into the hot skillet, 3 pancakes at a time. Cook for 4 to 5 minutes, then flip with a spatula to brown the other side. The pancakes will rise in the pan after flipping thanks to all that baking powder. Cook for an additional 3 to 5 minutes. Keep them warm while you make the next batch (see Ann's Tips, below).

5. Drizzle more butter over the skillet, rub in with the reserved paper towel, and make the next batch. Add a little more melted butter if needed. Repeat with the remaining batter. Eat dotted with a little butter and the peaches and blueberries in their syrup spooned on top.

Ann's Tips

· ✿ ·

In the winter, make a quick compote in the microwave with frozen fruit and 1 tablespoon of maple syrup; or instead of a peach, dice a fresh Bartlett pear and toss in the syrup as per the recipe.

If you want to make these pancakes but don't have buttermilk on hand, take a cup of milk and simply add either 1 teaspoon of lemon juice or a pinch of cream of tartar to it and let sit for 5 minutes while you pull together the other ingredients. This will lightly sour the milk, adding the acidity the recipe needs.

To keep the pancakes warm between batches, I put a heatproof plate over a pan of gently simmering water, top it with folded paper towels, and pop the pancakes between the sheets—where you might prefer still to be—while I cook the remaining pancakes.

Resources

Unless you live in a major city, it's not always easy to get the help or information you need to get through cancer treatment. There is a lot of unfiltered information about food and cancer on the Internet. Some of it is interesting and relevant, but some of it is downright dangerous. Listed here are some of the organizations that offer scientifically proven, reliable information about all types of cancer. From them you can get useful tips and advice, and find online support groups or programs.

THE AMERICAN CANCER SOCIETY (ACS)

Look for the latest on cancer research and nutrition info. For more than one hundred years, the American Cancer Society has worked relentlessly to save lives and create a world with less cancer. They help people stay well and get well, find cures, and fight against cancer. www.cancer.org

THE AMERICAN INSTITUTE FOR CANCER RESEARCH (AICR)

This is my favorite resource for dietary and lifestyle guidelines for cancer patients and caregivers. By funding research, interpreting evidence, and educating the public about the results, AICR is helping Americans realize that it's never too early or too late to make choices that protect against cancer. www.aicr.org

NATIONAL CANCER INSTITUTE (NCI)

The NCI, established under the National Cancer Institute Act of 1937, is the federal government's principal agency for cancer research and training. www.cancer.gov

THE CLEVELAND CLINIC

A nonprofit multispecialty academic medical center that integrates clinical and hospital care with research and education. They have useful information about different cancers and treatment protocols. http://my.clevelandclinic.org

THE MAYO CLINIC

The Mayo Clinic is a nonprofit worldwide leader in medical care, research, and education for people from all walks of life. Their website offers great nutrition information. www.mayoclinic.org

CANCERCARE

CancerCare is the leading national organization dedicated to providing free professional support services including counseling, support groups, educational workshops, publications, and financial assistance to anyone affected by cancer. www.cancercare.org

GILDA'S CLUB AND THE CANCER SUPPORT COMMUNITY

Gilda's Club offers free comprehensive cancer programs that include support groups, educational lectures, and workshops for everyone impacted by cancer—men, women, teens, and children—at their clubhouses throughout the country. Gilda's Club is represented nationally by the Cancer Support Community, an international nonprofit that ensures the empowerment of people impacted by cancer. Look on their websites to find your nearest Gilda's clubhouse or your local Cancer Support Community chapter or group. www.gildasclubnyc.org and www.cancersupportcommunity.org

STUPID CANCER

If you are a cancer patient or survivor under forty, your problems are different. Stupid Cancer can help you. A 501(c)(3) nonprofit organization, it is the largest charity that comprehensively addresses young adult cancer through advocacy, research, support, outreach, awareness, mobile health, and social media. Their innovative, award-winning, and evidence-based programs and services serve as a global bullhorn to propel the young adult cancer movement forward.

USEFUL INFORMATION ON GETTING THE BEST
THERE IS IN THE FOOD WE BUY

The Environmental Working Group (EWG): Creators of the Dirty Dozen and the Clean 15—the fruits and vegetables that we should buy organic, and the ones we don't need to. The Environmental Working Group is an American environmental organization that specializes in research and advocacy in the areas of agriculture and especially in toxic chemicals, including those found in pesticides, household products, and cosmetics. www.ewg.org

Monterey Bay Aquarium's Seafood Watch Sustainable Seafood App: Their app recommends seafood to buy or avoid, helping you select items that are fished or farmed in ways that have less impact on the environment. Get their recommendations and reports and learn the stories behind your seafood. www.seafood watch.org or (831) 648-7980

Animal Welfare Approved (AWA): a food label for meat and dairy products that come from farm animals raised to the highest animal welfare and environmental standards. http://animalwelfareapproved.org

Certified Humane: Look for their label.

Humane Farm Animal Care (HFAC): an international nonprofit certification organization dedicated to improving the lives of farm animals in food production from birth through slaughter. The goal of the program is to improve the lives of farm animals by driving consumer demand for kinder and more responsible farm animal practices. http://certifiedhumane.org

FINDING SPECIALTY FOODS

If you find it difficult to track down some of the ingredients we use in the recipes at your local markets, the Internet makes it easy to get most of these items delivered right to your door.

For all things South Asian or Middle Eastern, from whole and ground spices, to bulk nuts, to different types of rice, beans, and lentils:

 Kalustyan's (www.kalustyans.com)
 Amazon (smile.amazon.com)

For spices only:

 Penzeys Spices (www.penzeys.com)

Not all of us have a Whole Foods or a Trader Joe's nearby. If you can't find Asian foods like miso, kimchi, rice vinegar, soy sauce, and tofu in the macrobiotic section at your local market or health food store, you can find all of these things at:

 Amazon (smile.amazon.com)
 Asian Food Grocer (www.asianfoodgrocer.com)
 Mitsuwa Marketplace (www.mitsuwa.com)

Index